Medical
Coding Workbook

for Physician Practices and Facilities

2018–2019 Edition

Cynthia Newby, CPC, CPC-P

Principal, Chestnut Hill Enterprises, Inc.

McGraw Hill Education

MEDICAL CODING WORKBOOK FOR PHYSICIAN PRACTICES AND FACILITIES 2018–2019 Edition, EIGHTH EDITION

Published by McGraw-Hill Education, 2 Penn Plaza, New York, NY 10121. Copyright © 2018 by McGraw-Hill Education. All rights reserved. Printed in the United States of America. Previous editions © 2015, 2012, and 2010. No part of this publication may be reproduced or distributed in any form or by any means, or stored in a database or retrieval system, without the prior written consent of McGraw-Hill Education, including, but not limited to, in any network or other electronic storage or transmission, or broadcast for distance learning.

Some ancillaries, including electronic and print components, may not be available to customers outside the United States.

This book is printed on acid-free paper.

1 2 3 4 5 6 7 8 9 LMN 21 20 19 18 17

ISBN 978-1-259-63002-6
MHID 1-259-63002-1

Chief Product Officer, SVP, Products & Markets: *G. Scott Virkler*
Vice President, General Manager, Products & Markets: *Marty Lange*
Vice President, Content Design & Delivery: *Besty Whalen*
Managing Director: *Thomas Timp*
Brand Manager: *William Mulford*
Product Developer: *Michelle Gaseor*
Marketing Manager: *Roxan Kinsey*
Director, Content Design & Delivery: *Linda Avenarius*
Program Manager: *Angie FitzPatrick*
Content Project Manager: *Mary Jane Lampe*
Buyer: *Laura Fuller*
Cover Design: *Studio Montage*
Content Licensing Specialist: *Brianna Kirschbaum*
Cover Image: © *Brand X/Superstock*
Compositor: *Aptara®, Inc.*
Printer: *LSC Communications*

Source of CPT Codes: CPT only © 2017 American Medical Association. All rights reserved.

All credits appearing on page or at the end of the book are considered to be an extension of the copyright page.

CPT five-digit codes, nomenclature, and other data are copyright © 2017, American Medical Association. All rights reserved. No fee schedules, basic unit, relative values, or related listings are included in CPT. The AMA assumes no liability for the data contained herein.

CPT codes are based on CPT 2017.

HCPCS codes are based on HCPCS 2017.

ICD-10-CM codes are based on ICD-10-CM 2017.

mheducation.com/highered

Brief Contents

Contents

To the Student

Expertise in working with the HIPAA-mandated code sets found in ICD-10-CM, CPT®, and HCPCS is the baseline for correct coding. The diagnosis and procedure codes that physician practices and hospitals report to payers must be properly assigned based on current classifications. Equally important is knowing how to assign and report codes in compliance with government and other regulations such as HIPAA. To avoid potential billing fraud, the diagnoses on each medical insurance claim must support the medical necessity of the procedures. In addition to this code linkage, the reported services and procedures must be correctly documented in the patient medical record.

With many thousands of diagnosis and procedure codes to select from, however, developing coding expertise cannot be based on memorization or on trial and error! Rather, coders must understand the structure and conventions used in ICD-10-CM, CPT, and HCPCS, and know the guidelines for applying the codes. Coders also need to know the principles that underlie rules and regulations for compliant claims.

Medical Coding Workbook for Physician Practices and Facilities builds coding expertise by providing extensive practice in code selection. It is designed to be used in conjunction with ICD-10-CM, CPT, and HCPCS. ICD-10-PCS is required for Section 8 of Part 3. A medical dictionary and other medical references will also be helpful as you work through the coding exercises.

The workbook has three sections: Part 1, ICD-10-CM; Part 2, CPT and HCPCS, and Part 3, Auditing Linkage and Compliance. The exercises in the parts follow the structure of the coding references. Each set of exercises also presents Coding Tips to extend your knowledge of coding principles.

Because of the importance of correct coding, many medical coders seek certification as professional coders from organizations such as the American Academy of Professional Coders and the American Health Information Management Association. Certification examinations are taken after the coder has had both coding education and work experience. The Coding Quizzes in *Medical Coding Workbook for Physician Practices and Facilities* introduce you to the format of these exams and are useful in helping you build coding skill.

To the Instructor

Medical Coding Workbook for Physician Practices and Facilities is designed for use by students who have a basic understanding of medical coding from introductory instruction. For example, the McGraw-Hill text *Medical Insurance* (by Valerius et al.) is designed for medical insurance courses and devotes three chapters to physician practice coding. In the text, students learn the structure and conventions of ICD-10-CM and CPT and HCPCS and the correct process for selecting codes, as well as types of coding errors to be avoided.

New for the 2018–2019 Edition

Key changes for the new edition include updates to all codes for the 2017 code sets and new exercises covering major new codes.

Answers to the exercises in this workbook with coding rationales that show the pathways to correct codes are available for instructors using *Medical Coding Workbook for Physician Practices and Facilities* at the book's Online Learning Center, www.mhhe.com/codingwkbk8e. The Answer Key is also posted to the Online Learning Center for Valerius, *Medical Insurance*. Your McGraw-Hill sales representative can provide you with access.

The technical reviewers over many editions have offered invaluable assistance in reviewing the exercises, answers, and coding tips for accuracy. The reviewers and I hope that we have been correct in our work. Any errors, however, are the author's responsibility. You are encouraged to report these to the publisher so that corrections can be made.

Introducing SelectCoder Curriculum!

You know that the future starts with education, and the new SelectCoder Curriculum is designed specifically for the coding student. Using the same user-friendly, online medical coding and billing application offered in the market today through SelectCoder, the curriculum version presents all of the essential coding information that students and faculty need.

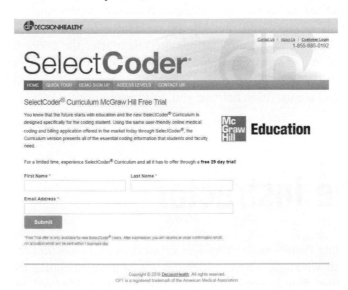

SelectCoder Curriculum is offered to students and faculty for up to one year. With your subscription, you'll receive:

- Documentation Finder™: Clinician documentation references to make correct ICD-10 code selection.
- Plain English descriptions: Easy-to-understand guidance to code quicker and process more claims.

- Coder's Pink Sheet™ specialty articles, tips, and expert guidance to bridge code understanding in the real-world provider setting.
- Official AMA CPT® coding guidelines: Assemble ICD-10 codes with ease to ensure coding accuracy and regulatory compliance.
- CPT® HCPCS, ICD-9-CM, ICD-10-CM, and modifiers: Quickly search to find codes, descriptions and instructional notes.
- ICD-10-CM mappings: Connect ICD-9 to ICD-10 smoothly with code mappings and unmatched expert guidance you can tap into as you code.
- CPT crosslinks: Procedure crosslinks to ICD-10, HCPCS, and modifiers for complete claims coding.
- LCD/NCD policies, covered ICD-9-CM/ICD-10-CM and validation tool: Up to date MAC-specific coverage policies with the click of a mouse.
- Medicare CCI edits with code bundling validation: At-a-glance code pair restrictions.
- Fees, RVUs for facility and non-facility: Reveal reimbursement impact of code choices.

Curriculum pricing includes a subscription for one year with a 50 percent discount off the regular price when you use **promo code MCGGRAD**. For a limited time, experience SelectCoder and all it has to offer through a free 29-day trial! Simply visit www.selectcoder.com/mcgrawhill to register today.

To learn more about SelectCoder Curriculum, visit www.selectcoder.com/mcgrawhill.

CPT® is a registered trademark of the American Medical Association.

Acknowledgments

Suggestions have been received from faculty and students throughout the country. This is vital feedback that is relied upon with each edition. Each of those who have offered comments and suggestions has our thanks.

The efforts of many people are needed to develop and improve a product. Among these people are the reviewers and consultants who point out areas of concern, cite areas of strength, and make recommendations for change. In this regard, the following people provided feedback that was enormously helpful in preparing the new edition.

- Ellen Anderson, M.Ad.Ed, RHIA, CCS, College of Lake County
- Nikita Carr, CPC, ICD-10 Corporate Trainer
- Deborah S. Gilbert, RHIA, MBA, CMA, Dalton State College
- April Green, CPC, San Joaquin Valley College
- Susan D. Hernandez, San Joaquin Valley College
- Jennifer Lame, MPH, RHIT, Southwest Wisconsin Technical College
- Deborah Montgomery, MBA, New River Community and Technical College
- Rolando Russell, MBA, RHIA, CPC, CPAR, Ultimate Medical Academy
- Karen S. Saba, CPC, CPC-I, Spokane Community College
- Barbara Temple, RHIT, CCS, CPC, CDIP, University of Arkansas Medical Sciences
- Kathy Ware, MCLS, RHIT, CPC, CPB, CPC-I, Lord Fairfax Community College

ACKNOWLEDGMENTS FROM THE AUTHOR

To the students and instructors who use this book, your feedback and suggestions have made the *Coding Workbook* a better learning tool for all.

I especially want to thank the editorial team at McGraw-Hill—Thomas Timp, Bill Mulford, and Michelle Gaseor—for their enthusiastic support. This book's continued success also owes much to the tireless efforts of Roxan Kinsey, Executive Marketing Manager.

The CPTS staff—content project manager Mary Jane Lampe and buyer Laura Fuller—was also outstanding in their efforts.

Thanks to this enthusiastic and dedicated team for making the revision process a seamless one!

Cynthia Newby, CPC, CPC-P

Part 1 ICD-10-CM

P art 1 of the *Medical Coding Workbook for Physician Practices and Facilities* begins with a brief review of ICD-10-CM coding basics as an overview/refresher to the coding exercises and quiz that follow. Study these points and be familiar with the coding terminology before completing the exercises and the quiz.

Note that the exercises begin by providing practice using external cause codes and nonillness factors (Z codes). This approach provides the training needed to then assign these codes as appropriate along with codes from Chapters 1–19 for diseases, illnesses, and injuries.

The exercises, which cover every chapter of ICD-10-CM, are designed to build your skill in applying the coding guidelines. Each chapter first overviews the purpose of the codes and then provides a coding tip or tips that explain important diagnostic coding rules, processes, or information. Some of these tips apply to a particular ICD-10-CM chapter and others apply globally.

After completion of all the exercises in this part, you will know how to apply guidelines concerning

- Z codes—primary or supplementary
- External cause codes—a supplementary classification
- Seventh-character extensions
- "Includes" notes
- The Neoplasm Table

- Multiple lymph node sites
- "Excludes" notes
- Coding for diabetes mellitus
- Coding for overweight and obesity
- The abbreviations NEC and NOS
- "Code first underlying disease" instruction
- Ischemic heart disease
- Hypertension
- Chronic versus acute conditions
- Digestive system combination codes
- Pressure ulcers
- Site and laterality
- Pathological versus traumatic fractures
- Chronic kidney disease (CKD)
- Mothers' conditions
- Normal pregnancy
- Infants' conditions
- Congenital anomalies and patients' ages
- Combination codes for typical symptoms
- HIV codes
- Laterality, healing stage, and episode of care for injuries
- Defaults for fracture coding
- Burns
- Poisoning, adverse effects, and underdosing

Review of ICD-10-CM

Learning Outcomes

After reviewing the basic instructions for coding with ICD-10-CM, you should be able to:

1-1 Discuss the purpose of ICD-10-CM.

1-2 Describe the organization of ICD-10-CM.

1-3 Summarize the structure, content, and key conventions of the Alphabetic Index.

1-4 Summarize the structure, content, and key conventions of the Tabular List.

1-5 Discuss the types of rules that are provided in the *ICD-10-CM Official Guidelines for Coding and Reporting*.

1-6 Briefly describe the content of Chapters 1 through 21 of the Tabular List.

1-7 List the steps in the process of assigning correct ICD-10-CM diagnosis codes.

Key Terms

acute
Alphabetic Index
category
chief complaint (CC)
chronic
code
coexisting condition (comorbidity)
combination code
convention
default code
diagnostic statement
eponym
etiology
excludes 1

excludes 2
exclusion note
external cause code
first-listed code
GEM
ICD-10-CM
ICD-10-CM Official Guidelines for Coding and Reporting
inclusion note
Index to External Causes
laterality
main term
manifestation
NEC (not elsewhere classified)

Neoplasm Table
nonessential modifier
NOS (not otherwise specified)
placeholder character (X)
primary diagnosis
principal diagnosis
sequelae
seventh-character extension
subcategory
subterm
Table of Drugs and Chemicals
Tabular List
Z code

Introduction to ICD-10-CM

Scientists and medical researchers have long gathered information from hospital records about patients' illnesses and causes of death. In place of written descriptions of the many different symptoms and conditions people have, standardized diagnosis codes have been developed for recording them. A coding system provides an accurate way to collect statistics to keep people healthy and to plan for needed health care resources, as well as to record morbidity (disease) and mortality (death) data.

Diagnosis codes are used to report patients' conditions on claims. Physicians determine the diagnosis. The physicians, medical coders, insurance/billing specialists, or medical assistants may be responsible for assigning the codes for those diagnoses. Expertise in diagnostic coding requires knowledge of medical terminology, pathophysiology, and anatomy, as well as experience in correctly applying the guidelines for assigning codes.

Under HIPAA, the diagnosis codes that must be used in the United States as of October 1, 2015, are based on the *International Classification of Diseases (ICD),* Tenth Revision. ICD-10 lists diseases and codes according to a system copyrighted by the World Health Organization of the United Nations. ICD has been revised a number of times since the coding system was first developed more than a hundred years ago.

ICD-10 has been the classification used by the federal government to categorize mortality data from death certificates since 1999. An expanded version of this tenth revision was published prior to the mandated compliance date for review by the healthcare community. A committee of healthcare professionals from various organizations and specialties prepared this version, which is called the ICD-10's *Clinical Modification,* or **ICD-10-CM.** It is used to code and classify morbidity data from patient medical records, physician offices, and surveys conducted by the National Center for Health Statistics (NCHS). Codes in ICD-10-CM describe conditions and illnesses more precisely than does the World Health Organization's ICD-10 because the codes are intended to provide a more complete picture of patients' conditions.

Code Makeup

An ICD-10-CM diagnosis code has between three and seven alphanumeric characters. The system is built on categories for diseases, injuries, and symptoms. A category has three characters. Most categories have subcategories of either four- or five-character codes. Valid codes themselves are either three, four, five, six, or seven characters in length, depending on the number of subcategories provided. For example, the code for the first visit for a closed and displaced fracture of the right tibial spine requires seven characters:

> Category S82 **Fracture of lower leg, including ankle**
> > Subcategory S82.1 **Fracture of upper end of tibia**
> > > Subcategory S82.11 **Fracture of tibial spine**
> > > > Code S82.111 **Displaced fracture of right tibial spine**
> > > > > Code S82.111A **Displaced fracture of tibial spine, initial encounter for closed fracture**

This variable structure enables coders to assign the most specific diagnosis that is documented in the patient medical record. A sixth character is more specific than the fourth or fifth characters, and the seventh-character extension can provide additional specific information about the health-related condition. When they are available for assignment in the ICD-10-CM code set, sixth and seventh characters are not optional; they must be used. For example, Centers for Medicare and Medicaid Services (CMS) rules state that a Medicare claim will be rejected when the most specific code available is not used.

Updates

The National Center for Health Statistics and CMS release ICD-10-CM updates called *addenda.* Since ICD-10-CM is still fairly new, it can be anticipated that more changes will be made over the next few years. The major new, invalid, and revised codes are posted on the appropriate websites, such as the NCHS and CMS websites.

New codes must be used as of the date they go into effect, and invalid (deleted) codes must not be used. The U.S. Government Printing Office (GPO) publishes the official ICD-10-CM on the Internet and in CD-ROM format every year. Various commercial publishers include the updated codes in annual coding books that are printed soon after the updates are released. The current reference must always be in use for the date of service of the encounter being coded.

> *ICD-10-CM Updates:*
> > www.cdc.gov/nchs/icd/icd10cm.htm
> > www.cms.gov/ICD10

Conversion from Previous Diagnosis Code Set

ICD-10-CM, as the name implies, is the tenth version of the diagnostic code set. The previous version is called ICD-9-CM. In rare situations, coders will be called upon to research an ICD-9-CM code. Perhaps an old claim has resurfaced, or an audit forces a review of pre-2015 codes that were reported. Workers' compensation (WC) claims may also specify a non-ICD-10-CM code set, because WC is not regulated by HIPAA law and therefore is not required to use ICD-10-CM.

The federal government has prepared **GEMs,** an acronym that stands for general equivalence mappings. Although imperfect, GEMs may be helpful in these situations. Both files of equivalent codes and a conversion tool may be located via an Internet search. Particularly useful is the translator tool located on the American Association of Professional Coders (AAPC) website.

> *ICD-10-CM to ICD-9-CM Conversion Tool:*
>   www.aapc.com/icd-10/codes/index.aspx

Note that confusion may result if the coder mixes up the ICD-9-CM codes that start with the capital letter E with those in ICD-10-CM that also start with E. There are a number of codes that are the same in both systems but have different meaning. Being clear on which system is in use will help the coder avoid these problems.

Organization of ICD-10-CM

ICD-10-CM has two major parts:

ICD-10-CM Index to Diseases and Injuries: The major section of this part, known as the **Alphabetic Index,** provides an index of the disease descriptions in the second major part, the Tabular List. Many descriptions are listed in more than one manner.

ICD-10-CM Tabular List of Diseases and Injuries: The **Tabular List** is made up of 21 chapters of disease descriptions and their codes.

ICD-10-CM's first part also has three additional sections that provide resources for researching correct codes:

ICD-10-CM Neoplasm Table: The **Neoplasm Table** provides code numbers for neoplasms by anatomical site and is divided by the description of the neoplasm.

ICD-10-CM Table of Drugs and Chemicals: The **Table of Drugs and Chemicals** provides an index in table format of drugs and chemicals that are listed in the Tabular List.

ICD-10-CM Index to External Causes: The **Index to External Causes** provides an index of all the external causes of diseases and injuries that are listed in the related chapter of the Tabular List.

The process of assigning ICD-10-CM codes begins with the physician's **diagnostic statement,** which contains the medical term describing the condition for which a patient is receiving care. For each encounter, this medical documentation includes the main reason for the patient encounter. It may also provide descriptions of additional conditions or symptoms that have been treated or that are related to the patient's current illness.

In each part of ICD-10-CM, **conventions,** which are typographic techniques that provide visual guidance for understanding information, help coders understand the rules and select the right code. The primary rule is that both the Alphabetic Index and the Tabular List are used sequentially to pick a code. The coder first locates the description/code in the Alphabetic Index and then verifies the proposed code selection by turning to the Tabular List and studying its entries.

This process must be followed when assigning all codes. A code followed by a hyphen in the Alphabetic Index is a clear reminder of this rule. The hyphen means that the coder will need to drill down to select the right code. For example, the index entry for otitis media is H66.9-. The coder turns to the Tabular List and reviews these entries:

H66.90 Otitis media, unspecified, unspecified ear

H66.91 Otitis media, unspecified, right ear

H66.92 Otitis media, unspecified, left ear

H66.93 Otitis media, unspecified, bilateral

Based on the documentation, one of these must be selected for compliant coding; just H66.9 is not sufficient.

The Alphabetic Index

The Alphabetic Index contains all the medical terms in the Tabular List classifications. For some conditions, it also lists common terms that are not found in the Tabular List. The index is organized by the *condition*, not by the body part (anatomical site) in which it occurs.

> The term *wrist fracture* is located by looking under *fracture, traumatic* (the condition) and then, below it, *wrist* (the location), rather than under *wrist* to find *fracture*.

Main Terms, Subterms, and Nonessential Modifiers

The assignment of the correct code begins with looking up the medical term that describes the patient's condition based on the diagnostic statement. Figure 1-1 illustrates the format of the Alphabetic Index. Each **main term** appears in boldface type and is followed by its **default code,** the one most frequently associated with it. For example, if the diagnostic statement is "the patient presents with blindness," the main term *blindness* is located in the Alphabetic Index (see Figure 1-1); the default code shown is H54.0.

Below the main term, any **subterms** with their codes appear. Subterms are essential in the selection of correct codes. They may show the **etiology** of the disease—its cause or origin—or describe a particular type or body site for the main term. For example, the main term *blindness* in Figure 1-1 includes 21 subterms, each indicating a different etiology or type—such as color blindness—for that condition.

Any **nonessential modifiers** for main terms or subterms are shown in parentheses on the same line. Nonessential modifiers are supplementary terms that are not essential to the selection of the correct code. They help point to the correct term, but they do not have to appear in the physician's diagnostic statement for the coder to correctly select the code. In Figure 1-1, for example, any of the

```
Blind (see also Blindness)                              mind R48.8
    bronchus (congenital) Q32.4                         night H53.60
    loop syndrome K90.2                                     abnormal dark adaptation curve H53.61
        congenital Q43.8                                    acquired H53.62
    sac, fallopian tube (congenital) Q50.6                  congenital H53.63
    spot, enlarged—see Defect, visual field, localized,     specified type NEC H53.69
        scotoma, blind spot area                            vitamin A deficiency E50.5
    tract or tube, congenital NEC—see Artresia, by site one eye (other eye normal) H54.40
Blindness (acquired) (congenital) (both eyes) H54.0         left (normal vision on right) H54.42
    blast S05.8x-                                               low vision on right H54.12
    color—see Deficiency, color vision                      low vision, other eye H54.10
    concussion S05.8x-                                      right (normal vision on left) H54.41
    cortical H47.619                                            low vision on left H54.11
        left brain H47.612                              psychic R48.8
        right brain H47.611                             river B73.01
    day H53.11                                          snow—see Photokeratitis
    due to injury (current episode) S05.9-              sun, solar—see Retinopathy, solar
        sequelae—code to injury with seventh           transient—see Disturbance, vision, subjective,
            character S                                     loss, transient
    eclipse (total)—see Retinopathy, solar              traumatic (current episode) S05.9-
    emotional (hysterical) F44.6                        word (developmental) F81.0
    face H53.16                                             acquired R48.0
    hysterical F44.6                                        secondary to organic lesion R48.0
    legal (both eyes) (USA definition) H54.8
```

Figure 1-1   Format of the Alphabetic Index

supplementary terms *acquired, congenital,* and *both eyes* may modify the main term in the diagnostic statement, such as "the patient presents with blindness acquired in childhood," or none of these terms may appear.

Common Terms

Many terms appear more than once in the Alphabetic Index. Often, the term in common use is listed, as well as the accepted medical terminology. For example, there is an entry for *flu*, with a cross-reference to *influenza*.

Eponyms

An **eponym** (pronounced ĕp'-∩-nim) is a condition (or a procedure) named for a person, such as the physician who discovered or invented it; some are named for patients. An eponym is usually listed both under that name and under the main term *disease* or *syndrome*. For example, Hodgson's disease appears as a subterm under *disease* and as a key term. The Alphabetic Index is the guide for coding other syndromes, such as battered child syndrome or HIV infection; if the syndrome is not identified, its manifestations are assigned codes.

Indention: Turnover Lines

If the main term or subterm is too long to fit on one line, as is often the case when many nonessential modifiers appear, turnover (or carryover) lines are used. Turnover lines are always indented farther to the right than are subterms. It is important to read carefully to distinguish a turnover line from a subterm line. For example, under the main term *blindness* (Figure 1-1) and the subterm *transient*, the information under "*see*" is long enough to require a turnover line. Without close attention, it is possible to confuse a turnover entry with a subterm.

Cross-References

Some entries use cross-references. If the cross-reference *see* appears after a main term, the coder *must* look up the term that follows the word *see* in the index. The *see* reference means that the main term where the coder first looked is not correct; another category must be used. In Figure 1-1, for example, to code the subterm *snow* under *blind*, the term *Photokeratitis* must be found.

See also, another type of cross-reference, points the coder to additional, related index entries. *See also category* indicates that the coder should review the additional categories that are mentioned. For example, in Figure 1-1, the *see also* note at *Blind* directs the coder to check subterm *snow* under *blindness* as well.

The Abbreviations NEC and NOS

Not elsewhere classified, or **NEC,** appears with a term when there is no code that is specific for the condition. This abbreviation means that no code matches the exact situation. For example:

Hemorrhage, eye NEC H57.8

Another abbreviation, **NOS,** or **not otherwise specified,** means *unspecified.* This term or abbreviation indicates that the code to be located in the Tabular List should be used when a condition is not completely described in the medical record. For example:

Enteritis, bacillary NOS A03.9

Multiple Codes, Connecting Words, and Combination Codes

Some conditions may require two codes, one for the etiology and a second for the **manifestation,** the disease's typical signs, symptoms, or secondary processes. This requirement is indicated when two codes, the second in brackets, appear after a term:

Pneumonia in rheumatic fever I00 [*J17*]

This entry indicates that the diagnostic statement "pneumonia in rheumatic fever" requires two codes, one for the etiology (rheumatic fever, I00) and one for the manifestation (pneumonia, J17). The use of brackets in the Alphabetic Index around a code means that it cannot be the **first-listed code** in coding this diagnostic statement; these codes are listed after the codes for the etiology.

The use of connecting words, such as *due to, during, following,* and *with,* may also indicate the need for two codes or for a single code that covers both conditions. For example, the main term below is followed by a *due to* subterm:

Cramp(s), muscle, R25.2
    due to immersion T75.1

When the Alphabetic Index indicates the possible need for two codes, the Tabular List entry is used to determine whether in fact they are needed. In some cases, a **combination code** describing both the etiology and the manifestation is available instead of two codes. For example:

Influenza due to identified novel influenza A virus with gastrointestinal manifestations J09.X3

Combination codes may also exist that classify two diagnoses or a diagnosis with an associated complication.

The Tabular List

The Tabular List received its name from the language of statistics; the word *tabulate* means to count, record, or list systematically. The diseases and injuries in the Tabular List are organized into chapters according to etiology, body system, or purpose. The organization of the Tabular List and the ranges of codes each part covers are shown in Table 1.1.

Table 1.1 ICD-10-CM Chapter Structure

Chapter	Code Range	Title
1	A00–B99	Certain infectious and parasitic diseases
2	C00–D49	Neoplasms
3	D50–D89	Diseases of the blood and blood-forming organs and certain disorders involving the immune mechanism
4	E00–E89	Endocrine, nutritional and metabolic diseases
5	F01–F99	Mental, behavioral and neurodevelopmental disorders
6	G00–G99	Diseases of the nervous system
7	H00–H59	Diseases of the eye and adnexa
8	H60–H95	Diseases of the ear and mastoid process
9	I00–I99	Diseases of the circulatory system
10	J00–J99	Diseases of the respiratory system
11	K00–K95	Diseases of the digestive system
12	L00–L99	Diseases of the skin and subcutaneous tissue
13	M00–M99	Diseases of the musculoskeletal system and connective tissue
14	N00–N99	Diseases of the genitourinary system
15	O00–O9A	Pregnancy, childbirth and the puerperium
16	P00–P96	Certain conditions originating in the perinatal period
17	Q00–Q99	Congenital malformations, deformations and chromosomal abnormalities
18	R00–R99	Symptoms, signs and abnormal clinical and laboratory findings, not elsewhere classified
19	S00–T88	Injury, poisoning and certain other consequences of external causes
20	V00–Y99	External causes of morbidity
21	Z00–Z99	Factors influencing health status and contact with health services

Categories, Subcategories, and Codes

Each Tabular List chapter is divided into categories, subcategories, and codes.

1. A **category** is a three-character alphanumeric code that covers a single disease or related condition. For example, the category L03 in Figure 1-2 covers cellulitis and acute lymphangitis.

2. A **subcategory** is a four- or five-character alphanumeric subdivision of a category. It provides a further breakdown of the disease to show its etiology, site, or manifestation. For example, the L03 category has six subcategories:

   L03.0 Cellulitis and acute lymphangitis of finger and toe
   L03.1 Cellulitis and acute lymphangitis of other parts of limb
   L03.2 Cellulitis and acute lymphangitis of face and neck
   L03.3 Cellulitis and acute lymphangitis of trunk
   L03.8 Cellulitis and acute lymphangitis of other sites
   L03.9 Cellulitis and acute lymphangitis, unspecified

3. A **code,** the smallest division, has either 3, 4, 5, 6, or 7 alphanumeric characters. For example, locate five- and six-character codes in Figure 1-2.

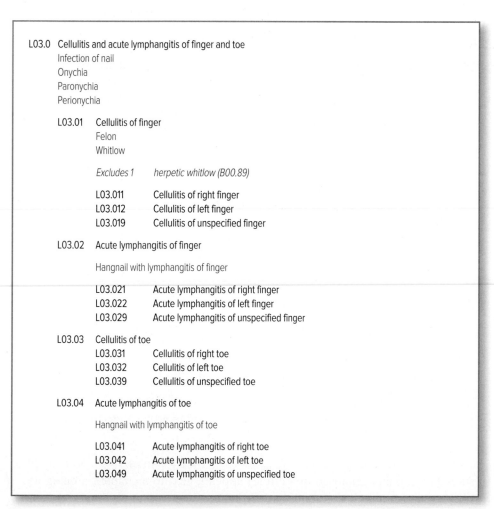

Figure 1-2 Format of Tabular List

Note that the first character in a code is always a letter. The complete alphabet, except for the letter U, is used. The second and third characters may be either numbers or letters, although currently the second character is usually (but not always) a number. A valid code has to have at least three characters. If it has more than that, a period is placed following the third character:

L03.112 Cellulitis of left axilla

Each character beyond the category level provides greater specificity to the code's meaning.

Placeholder Character Requirement

ICD-10-CM uses a **placeholder character** (also known as the "dummy placeholder") designated as "X" in some codes when a fifth-, sixth-, or seventh-digit character is required but the digit space to the left of that character is empty.

For example, the subcategory T46.1 Poisoning by, adverse effect of and underdosing of calcium-channel blockers, uses the *sixth* digit to describe whether the poisoning was accidental (unintentional), intentional self-harm, caused by assault, undetermined, or related to an adverse effect or underdosing. Since there is no fifth digit assigned, an X is used to hold that fifth space.

T46.1X2 Poisoning by calcium-channel blockers, intentional self-harm

Seventh-Character Extension

ICD-10-CM requires assigning a seventh character in some categories, usually to specify the sequence of the visit (for example, the initial encounter for the problem, the subsequent encounter for the problem, or sequela—the problem results from a previous disease or injury; the plural is *sequelae*). The **seventh-character extension** requirement is contained in a note at the start of the codes it covers. The seventh character must always be in position 7 of the alphanumeric code, so if the code is not at least six characters long, the placeholder character "X" must be used to fill that empty space.

For example, category S64, Injury of nerves at wrist and hand level, leads off with this note:

> The appropriate 7th character is to be added to each code from category S64.
> A   initial encounter
> D   subsequent encounter
> S   sequela

Subcategory S64.22, Injury of radial nerve at wrist and hand level of left arm, has no sixth digit but requires the seventh, so the correct code for an initial encounter would be:

S64.22XA Injury of radial nerve at wrist and hand level of left arm, initial encounter

Depending on the publisher of ICD-10-CM, a section mark (§) or other symbol (such as a number enclosed in a circle) appears next to a chapter, a category, a subcategory, or a code that requires a fifth, sixth, or seventh digit to be assigned. These are important reminders to assign the appropriate characters.

Inclusion Notes

Inclusion notes are headed by the word *includes* and refine the content of the category appearing above them. For example, after the three-digit category, L04, Acute lymphadenitis, the *inclusion* note states that the category includes abscess (acute) of the lymph nodes, except mesenteric, and acute lymphadenitis, except mesenteric.

Exclusion Notes

Exclusion notes are headed by the word *excludes* and indicate conditions that are not classifiable to the code above. Two types of exclusion notes are used. **Excludes 1** is used when two conditions could not exist together, such as an acquired and a congenital condition; it means "not coded here." **Excludes 2** means "not included here," but a patient could have both conditions at the same time. An example occurs in the category L04, again. This *excludes* note states that the category does not include enlarged lymph nodes, among other conditions. The note may also give the code(s) of the excluded condition(s).

Punctuation

Colons

A colon (:) indicates an incomplete term. One or more of the entries following the colon is required to make a complete term. Unlike terms in parentheses or brackets, when the colon is used, the diagnostic statement must include one of the terms after the colon to be assigned a code from the particular category. For example, the *excludes* note after the information for chorioretinal disorders is as follows:

> H32 Chorioretinal disorders in diseases classified elsewhere
> *Excludes 1: chorioretinitis (in):*
> *toxoplasmosis (acquired) (B58.01)*
> *tuberculosis (A18.53)*

For the *excludes* note to apply to *chorioretinitis*, "acquired toxoplasmosis" or "tuberculosis" must appear in the diagnostic statement.

Parentheses

Parentheses ( ) are used around descriptions that do not affect the code—that is, nonessential, supplementary terms. For example, the subcategory G24.1, Genetic torsion dystonia, is followed by the entry "Idiopathic (torsion) dystonia NOS."

Brackets

Brackets [ ] are used around synonyms, alternative wordings, or explanations. They have the same meaning as parentheses. For example, category E52 is described as "Niacin deficiency [pellagra]."

Abbreviations: NEC versus NOS

NEC and NOS are used in the Tabular List with the same meanings as in the Alphabetic Index.

Etiology/Manifestation Coding

The convention that addresses multiple codes for conditions that have both an underlying etiology and manifestations is indicated in the Tabular List by some phrases that contain instructions about the need for additional codes. The phrases point to situations in which more than one code is required. For example, a statement that a condition is "due to" or "associated with" may require an additional code.

Use Additional Code

The etiology code may be followed by the instruction *use an additional code* or a note saying the same thing. The order of the codes must be the same as shown in the Alphabetic Index: the etiology comes first, followed by the manifestation code.

Code First Underlying Disease

The instruction *code first underlying disease* (or similar wording) appears below a manifestation code that must not be used as a first-listed code. These codes are for symptoms only, never for causes. At times, a specific instruction is given, such as in this example:

> **F07 Personality and behavioral disorders due to known physiological condition**
> Code first the underlying physiological condition

Other "Use Additional Code" Requirements

The "use additional code" note also appears when ICD-10-CM requires assignment of codes for health factors such as tobacco use and alcohol use.

Laterality

The Tabular List provides a coding structure based on the concept of **laterality.** In ICD-10-CM, this is the idea that the classification system should capture the side of the body that is documented for a particular condition. The fourth, fifth, or sixth characters specify the affected side, such as right arm, left wrist, both eyes. (In general usage, laterality means a preference for one side of the body, like lefthandedness.) When the affected side of the condition is not known, an unspecified code is assigned. If the condition is documented as bilateral but there is no appropriate code for bilaterality (that is, both), two codes for the left and right sides are assigned.

ICD-10-CM Official Guidelines for Coding and Reporting

Assigning HIPAA-mandated diagnosis codes follows both the conventions that are incorporated in the Alphabetic Index/Tabular List as well as a separate set of rules called *ICD-10-CM Official Guidelines for Coding and Reporting*. Known as the *Official Guidelines,* these rules are developed by a group known as the four cooperating parties made up of CMS advisers and participants from the American Hospital Association (AHA), the American Health Information Management Association (AHIMA), and the National Center for Health Statistics (NCHS).

ICD-10-CM Official Guidelines
www.cdc.gov/nchs/icd/icd10cm.htm

The *Official Guidelines* have sections for general rules, inpatient (hospital) coding, and outpatient (physician office/clinic) coding:

- Section I, *Conventions, general coding guidelines, and chapter-specific guidelines,* first reviews the Alphabetic Index and Tabular List conventions and broad coding rules, and then discusses key topics affecting the use of codes in each of the 21 chapters.

- Section II, *Selection of Principal Diagnosis,* and Section III, *Reporting Additional Diagnoses*, explain the guidelines for establishing the diagnosis or diagnoses for inpatient cases.

- Section IV, *Diagnostic Coding and Reporting Guidelines for Outpatient Services*, explains the guidelines for establishing the diagnosis or diagnoses for all outpatient encounters.

Appendix A of this *Medical Coding Workbook* presents Section IV. The key points from this section can be summarized as follows:

1. Code the primary diagnosis first, followed by current coexisting conditions.
2. Code to the highest level of certainty.
3. Code to the highest level of specificity.

Code the Primary Diagnosis First, Followed by Current Coexisting Conditions

ICD-10-CM code for the **primary diagnosis** is listed first.

● EXAMPLE

Diagnostic Statement: Patient is an elderly female complaining of back pain. For the past five days, she has had signs of pyelonephritis, including urinary urgency, urinary incontinence, and back pain. Has had a little hematuria, but no past history of urinary difficulties.

Primary Diagnosis: N12 Pyelonephritis ●

After the first-listed diagnosis, additional codes may be used to describe all current documented coexisting conditions that must be actively managed because they affect patient treatment or that require treatment during the encounter. **Coexisting conditions (comorbidities)** may be related to the primary diagnosis, or they may involve a separate illness that the physician diagnoses and treats during the encounter.

● EXAMPLE

Diagnostic Statement: Patient, a forty-five-year-old male, presents for complete physical examination for an insurance certification. During the examination, patient complains of occasional difficulty hearing; wax is removed from the left ear canal.

Primary Diagnosis: Z02.6 Routine physical examination for insurance certification

Coexisting Condition: H61.22 Impacted cerumen, left ear ●

It is important to note that patients may have diseases or conditions that do not affect the encounter being coded. Some physicians add notes about previous conditions to provide an easy reference to a patient's history. Unless these conditions are directly involved with the patient's treatment, they are not considered in selecting codes. Also, conditions that were previously treated and no longer exist are not coded.

● EXAMPLE

Chart Note: Mrs. Mackenzie, whose previous encounter was for her regularly scheduled blood pressure check to monitor her hypertension, presents today with a new onset of psoriasis.

Primary Diagnosis: L40.9 Psoriasis, unspecified ●

Coding Acute versus Chronic Conditions

The reasons for patient encounters are often **acute** symptoms—generally, relatively sudden or severe problems. Acute conditions are coded with the specific code that is designated acute, if listed. Many patients, however, receive ongoing treatment for **chronic** conditions—those that continue over a long period of time or recur frequently. For example, a patient may need a regular injection for the management of rheumatoid arthritis. In such cases, the disease is coded and reported for as many times as the patient receives care for the condition.

In some cases, an encounter covers both an acute and a chronic condition. Some conditions do not have separate entries for both manifestations, so a single code applies. If both the acute and the chronic illnesses have codes, the acute code is listed first.

● EXAMPLE

Acute renal failure, unspecified N17.9

Chronic renal failure, unspecified N18.9 ●

Coding Sequelae

A **sequela** is a condition that remains after a patient's acute illness or injury has ended. Often called residual effects or late effects, some happen soon after the disease is over, and others occur later. The diagnostic statement may say:

- Due to an old . . . (for example, swelling due to old contusion of knee)
- Late . . . (for example, nausea as a late effect of radiation sickness)
- Due to a previous . . . (for example, abdominal mass due to a previous spleen injury)
- Traumatic (if not a current injury); including scarring or nonunion of a fracture (for example, malunion of fracture, left humerus)

In general, the main term *sequela* is followed by subterms that list the causes. Two codes are usually required. First reported is the code for the specific effect (such as muscle soreness), followed by the code for the cause (such as the late effect of rickets). The code for the acute illness that led to the sequela is never used with a code for the late effect itself.

Code to the Highest Level of Certainty

Diagnoses are not always established at a first encounter. Follow-up visits over time may be required before the physician determines a primary diagnosis. During this process, although possible diagnoses may appear in the physician's documentation as diagnostic work is progressing, these inconclusive diagnoses are not used to determine the first-listed codes reported for reimbursement of service fees.

Signs and Symptoms

Instead of inconclusive diagnoses, the specific signs and symptoms are coded and reported. A *sign* is an objective indication that can be evaluated by the physician, such as weight loss. A *symptom* is a subjective statement by the patient that cannot be confirmed during an examination, such as pain.

The following case provides an example of how symptoms and signs are coded:

● EXAMPLE

Diagnostic Statement: Middle-aged male presents with abdominal pain and weight loss. He had to return home from vacation due to acute illness. He has not been eating well because of a vague upper-abdominal pain. He denies nausea, vomiting. He denies changes in bowel habit or blood in stool. Physical examination revealed no abdominal tenderness.

Primary Diagnosis: R10.13 Abdominal pain, epigastric region

Coexisting Condition: R63.4 Abnormal weight loss ●

Suspected Conditions

Similarly, possible but not confirmed diagnoses, such as those preceded by "rule out," "suspected," "probable," or "likely," are not coded in the outpatient (physician practice) setting.

Note that in the inpatient setting, however, the guidance is different. For hospital coding, the first-listed diagnosis is referred to as the **principal diagnosis** and is defined as the condition established after study to be chiefly responsible for the admission. "After study" means at the patient's discharge from the facility. If a definitive condition has not been established, then, at discharge, the inpatient coder codes the condition that matches the planned course of treatment most closely as if it were established.

Coding the Reason for Surgery

Surgery is coded according to the diagnosis that is listed as the reason for the procedure. In some cases, the postoperative diagnosis is available and is different from the physician's primary diagnosis before the surgery. If so, the postoperative diagnosis is coded because it is the highest level of certainty available. For example, if an excisional biopsy is performed to evaluate mammographic breast lesions or a lump of unknown nature, and the pathology results show a malignant neoplasm, the diagnosis code describing the site and nature of the neoplasm is used.

Code to the Highest Level of Specificity

The more characters a code has, the more specific it becomes; the additional characters add to the clinical picture of the patient. Using the most specific code possible is referred to as coding to the highest level of specificity. In the following example, the most specific code has six characters.

Category L03 **Cellulitis and acute lymphangitis** (three characters)
    Subcategory L03.0 **Cellulitis and acute lymphangitis of finger and toe** (four characters)
        Subcategory L03.01 **Cellulitis of finger** (five characters)
        Code L03.011 **Cellulitis of right finger** (six characters)

Code L03.012 **Cellulitis of left finger** (six characters)
Code L03.019 **Cellulitis of unspecified finger** (six characters)

However, note that the last code, L03.019, is considered less specific than the other six-character codes, because it indicates that the affected finger is not known. Appropriate documentation should provide this level of detail.

Other (or Other Specified) versus Unspecified

In the Tabular List, the coder may need to choose between a code described as the core condition, *other* (or *other specified*) versus *unspecified*. For example:

L70.8 Other acne
L70.9 Acne, unspecified

If the documentation mentions a type or form of the condition that is not listed, the coder chooses "other," because a type is indicated but not found. If no type is mentioned, the documentation is not complete enough to assign a more specific code, and so the least-specific choice, "unspecified," is assigned. If there is no other versus unspecified coding option, select the "other specified" which in this situation represents both "other" and "unspecified."

Overview of ICD-10-CM Chapters

A00–B99 Certain Infectious and Parasitic Diseases

Codes in Chapter 1 of ICD-10-CM's Tabular List classify communicable infectious and parasitic diseases. Most categories describe a condition and the type of organism that causes it.

C00–D49 Neoplasms

Neoplasms are coded from Chapter 2 of ICD-10-CM. Neoplasms (tumors) are growths that arise from normal tissue. Note that this category does not include a diagnosis statement with the word *mass*, which is a separate main term. The Alphabetic Index also contains a Neoplasm Table that points to codes for neoplasms. The table lists the anatomical location in the first column. The next six columns relate to the behavior of the neoplasm.

D50–D89 Diseases of the Blood and Blood-Forming Organs and Certain Disorders Involving the Immune Mechanism

Codes in this brief ICD-10-CM chapter classify diseases of the blood and blood-forming organs, such as anemias and coagulation defects, as well as some immune mechanism deficiencies.

E00–E89 Endocrine, Nutritional and Metabolic Diseases

Codes in Chapter 4 of ICD-10-CM classify a variety of conditions. The most common disease in this chapter is diabetes mellitus, which is a progressive disease of either type 1 or type 2, the predominant disease.

F01–F99 Mental, Behavioral and Neurodevelopmental Disorders

Codes in Chapter 5 of ICD-10-CM classify the various types of mental disorders, including conditions of drug and alcohol dependency, Alzheimer's disease, schizophrenic disorders, and mood disturbances. Most psychiatrists use the terminology found in the *Diagnostic and Statistical Manual of Mental Disorders (DSM)* for diagnoses, but the coding follows ICD-10-CM.

G00–G99 Diseases of the Nervous System

Codes in Chapter 6 classify diseases of the central nervous system and the peripheral nervous system.

H00–H59 Diseases of the Eye and Adnexa

Codes in Chapter 7 classify diseases of the eye and adnexa.

H60–H95 Diseases of the Ear and Mastoid Process

Codes in Chapter 8 classify diseases of the ear and mastoid process.

I00–I99 Diseases of the Circulatory System

Because Chapter 9 addresses the circulatory system, which involves so many interrelated components, the disease process can create interrelated, complex conditions. The notes and *code also* instructions must be carefully observed to code circulatory diseases accurately.

J00–J99 Diseases of the Respiratory System

Codes in Chapter 10 of ICD-10-CM classify respiratory illnesses such as influenza, pneumonia, chronic obstructive pulmonary disease (COPD), and asthma. Pneumonia, a common respiratory infection, may be caused by one of a number of organisms. Many codes for pneumonia include the condition and the cause in a combination code, such as J15.21, pneumonia due to Staphylococcus aureus.

K00–K95 Diseases of the Digestive System

Codes in Chapter 11 of ICD-10-CM classify diseases of the digestive system. Codes are listed according to anatomical location, beginning with the oral cavity and continuing through the intestines, liver, and related organs.

L00–L99 Diseases of the Skin and Subcutaneous Tissue

Codes in ICD-10-CM's Chapter 12 classify skin infections, inflammations, and other diseases.

M00–M99 Diseases of the Musculoskeletal System and Connective Tissue

Codes in Chapter 13 of ICD-10-CM classify conditions of the bones and joints—arthropathies (joint disorders), dorsopathies (back disorders), rheumatism, pathological fractures, and other diseases. In this huge chapter, codes are provided for both site and laterality. The site represents the bone, joint, or muscle that is affected. Many codes cover conditions affecting multiple sites, such as osteoarthritis.

N00–N99 Diseases of the Genitourinary System

Codes in Chapter 14 of ICD-10-CM classify diseases of the male and female genitourinary (GU) systems, such as infections of the genital tract, renal disease, conditions of the prostate, and problems with the cervix, vulva, and breast.

(O00–O9A) Pregnancy, Childbirth and the Puerperium

Codes in Chapter 15 of ICD-10-CM classify conditions that are involved with pregnancy, childbirth, and the puerperium (the six-week period following delivery).

P00–P96 Certain Conditions Originating in the Perinatal Period

Codes in Chapter 16 of ICD-10-CM classify conditions of the fetus or the newborn infant, the neonate, up to 28 days after birth. These codes are assigned only to conditions of the infant, not of the mother.

Q00–Q99 Congenital Malformations, Deformations and Chromosomal Abnormalities

Codes in ICD-10-CM Chapter 17 classify anomalies, malformations, and diseases that exist at birth. Unlike acquired disorders, congenital conditions are either hereditary or due to influencing factors during gestation.

R00–R99 Symptoms, Signs and Abnormal Clinical and Laboratory Findings, Not Elsewhere Classified

Codes in this 18th chapter of ICD-10-CM classify patients' symptoms, signs, and ill-defined conditions for which a definitive diagnosis cannot be made. In physician practice (outpatient) coding, these codes are always used instead of coding "rule out," "probable," or "suspected" conditions.

S00–T88 Injury, Poisoning and Certain Other Consequences of External Causes

Codes in Chapter 19 of ICD-10-CM classify injuries and wounds (fractures, dislocations, sprains, strains, internal injuries, and traumatic injuries), burns, poisoning, and various consequences of external causes. Often, additional codes from Chapter 20 are used to identify the cause of the injury or poisoning.

The Table of Drugs and Chemicals in the Alphabetic Index lists, for each drug, codes for accidental poisoning, intentional poisoning, poisoning from assault or undetermined cause, adverse effects, and underdosing. *Adverse effects,* which are unintentional, harmful reactions to a proper dosage of a drug properly taken, are different from *poisoning,* which refers to the medical result of the incorrect use of a substance, or *underdosing,* taking less of a medication than is prescribed by a provider or the manufacturer.

Most categories in Chapter 19 need the seventh-character extension to capture one of these three episodes of care:

A for an initial encounter
D for a subsequent encounter
S for sequela

For example, ICD-10-CM code S31.623A, Laceration with foreign body of abdominal wall, right lower quadrant with penetration into peritoneal cavity, initial encounter, shows a seventh character used with a laceration code.

V00–Y99 External Causes of Morbidity

Codes in Chapter 20 of ICD-10-CM classify **external cause codes,** which report the cause of injuries from various environmental events, such as transportation accidents, falls, and fires. External cause codes are not used alone or as first-listed codes. They always supplement a code that identifies the injury or condition itself.

Many blocks of accident and injury codes in this chapter require additional external cause codes for

- The encounter (A = initial, D = subsequent, or S = sequela)
- The place of occurrence (category Y92)
- The activity (category Y93)
- The status (category Y99)

External cause codes are located by first using the third section of the Alphabetic Index, Index to External Causes. This index is organized by main terms describing the accident, circumstance, or event that caused the injury. Codes are verified in Chapter 20 of the Tabular List.

External cause codes are often used in collecting public health information. They capture cause, intent, place, and activity. As many external cause codes as are needed to describe these factors should be reported. Note, however, that these codes are not needed if the external cause and intent are already included in a code from another chapter.

Z00–Z99 Factors Influencing Health Status and Contact with Health Services

Chapter 21 contains **Z codes** that are used to report encounters for circumstances other than a disease or injury, such as factors influencing health status, and to describe the nature of a patient's contact with health services. There are two chief types:

- Reporting visits with healthy (or ill) patients who receive services other than treatments, such as annual checkups, immunizations, and normal childbirth. This use is coded by a Z code that identifies the service, such as:

  Z00.01 Encounter for general adult medical examination with abnormal findings

- Reporting encounters in which a problem not currently affecting the patient's health status needs to be noted, such as personal and family history. For example, a person with a family history of breast cancer is at higher risk for the disease, and a Z code is assigned as an additional code for screening codes to explain the need for a test or procedure, as is shown here:

  Z80.3 Family history of malignant neoplasm of breast

A Z code can be used as either a primary code for an encounter or as an additional code. It is researched in the same way as other codes, using the Alphabetic Index to point to the term's code and the Tabular List to verify it. The terms that indicate the need for Z codes, however, are not the same as other medical terms. They usually have to do with a reason for an encounter other than a disease or its

Table 1.2 Terminology Associated with Z Codes

Term	Example
Contact/exposure	Z20.1 Contact with and (suspected) exposure to tuberculosis
Contraception	Z30.01 Encounter for initial prescription of contraceptives
Counseling	Z31.5 Encounter for genetic counseling
Examination	Z00.110 Health examination for newborn under 8 days old
Fitting of	Z46.51 Encounter for fitting and adjustment of gastric lap band
Follow-up	Z08 Encounter for follow-up examination after completed treatment for malignant neoplasm
History (of)	Z92.23 Personal history of estrogen therapy
Screening/test	Z11.51 Encounter for screening for human papillomavirus (HPV)
Status	Z67.10 Type A blood, Rh positive
Supervision (of)	Z34.01 Encounter for supervision of normal first pregnancy, first trimester
Vaccination/inoculation	Z23 Encounter for immunization

complications. When found in diagnostic statements, the words listed in Table 1.2 often point to Z codes.

Coding Steps

The correct procedure for assigning accurate diagnosis codes has six steps, as shown in Figure 1-3.

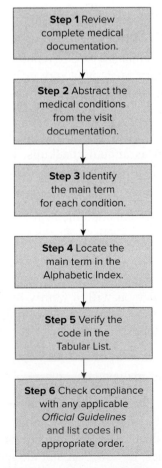

Step 1 Review complete medical documentation.

Step 2 Abstract the medical conditions from the visit documentation.

Step 3 Identify the main term for each condition.

Step 4 Locate the main term in the Alphabetic Index.

Step 5 Verify the code in the Tabular List.

Step 6 Check compliance with any applicable *Official Guidelines* and list codes in appropriate order.

Figure 1-3 Diagnosis Code Assignment Flowchart

Step 1:
Review Complete Medical Documentation

In outpatient settings, diagnosis coding begins with the patient's **chief complaint (CC)**. The chief complaint is the medical reason that the patient presents for the particular visit. This is documented in the patient's medical record. The physician then examines the patient and evaluates the condition or complaint, documenting the diagnosis, condition, problem, or other reason that the documentation shows as being chiefly responsible for the services that are provided. This primary diagnosis provides the main term to be coded first. Documentation will also mention any coexisting complaints that should be coded.

> If a patient has cancer, the disease is probably the patient's major health problem. However, if that patient sees the physician for an ear infection that is not related to the cancer, the primary diagnosis for that particular claim is the ear infection.

> A patient's examination might be documented as follows:

> CC: Diarrhea X 5 days with strong odor and mucus, abdominal pain and tenderness, no meds.
> Dx: Ulcerative colitis.

The notes mean that the patient has had symptoms for five days and has taken no medication. The chief complaint is noted after the abbreviation *CC*. The diagnosis, listed after the abbreviation *Dx*, is ulcerative colitis.

Assume that another patient's record indicates a history of heavy smoking and includes an x-ray report and notes such as these:

> CC: Hoarseness, pain during swallowing, dyspnea during exertion.
> Dx: Emphysema and laryngitis.

The physician listed emphysema, the major health problem, first; it is the primary diagnosis. Laryngitis is a coexisting condition that is being treated.

Step 2:
Abstract the Medical Conditions from the Visit Documentation

The code will be assigned based on the physician's diagnosis or diagnoses. This information may be located on the encounter form or elsewhere in the patient's medical record, such as in a progress note. For example, a medical record reads:

> CC: Chest and epigastric pain; feels like a burning inside. Occasional reflux. Abdomen soft, flat without tenderness. No bowel masses or organomegaly.
> Dx: Peptic ulcer.

The diagnosis is peptic ulcer.

Step 3:
Identify the Main Term for Each Condition

If needed, decide which is the main term or condition of the diagnosis. For example, in the diagnosis above, the main term or condition is *ulcer*. The word *peptic* describes what type of ulcer it is. Here are other examples:

Dx: Complete paralysis.

The main term is *paralysis*, and the supplementary term is *complete*.

Dx: Heart palpitation.

The main term is *palpitation*, and the supplementary term is *heart*.

Dx: Panner's disease.

This condition can be found in either of two ways: by looking up the main term *disease*, followed by *Panner's*, or by looking up *Panner's disease*.

Step 4:
Locate the Main Term in the Alphabetic Index

The main term for the patient's primary diagnosis is located in the Alphabetic Index. These guidelines should be observed in choosing the correct term:

• Use any supplementary terms in the diagnostic statement to help locate the main term.
• Read and follow any notes below the main term.
• Review the subterms to find the most specific match to the diagnosis.
• Read and follow any cross-references.
• Make note of a two-code (etiology and/or manifestation) indication.

Step 5:
Verify the Code in the Tabular List

The code for the main term is then located in the Tabular List. These guidelines are observed to verify the selection of the correct code:

• Read *includes* or *excludes* notes, checking back to see if any apply to the code's category, section, or chapter.
• Be alert for and follow instructions for fifth-digit requirements.
• Follow any instructions requiring the selection of additional codes (such as "code also" or "code first underlying disease"). This may require further research elsewhere in the Tabular List.
• List multiple codes in the correct order.

Step 6:
Check Compliance with Any Applicable *Official Guidelines* and List Codes in Appropriate Order

The final step is to review ICD-10-CM *Official Guidelines for Coding and Reporting* to check for applicable points. Coders should be sure not to include suspected conditions (for outpatient settings) and to report the primary diagnosis as the first-listed code, followed by any coexisting conditions and external source codes.

ICD-10-CM Terminology

Before working through the exercises that follow, be sure that you are familiar with the following key terms and their definitions.

acute illness or condition with severe symptoms and a short duration

Alphabetic Index part of ICD-CM-10 listing disease and injuries alphabetically with corresponding diagnosis codes

category three-character code for classifying a disease or condition

chief complaint (CC) patient's description of the symptoms or other reasons for seeking medical care

chronic illness or condition with a long duration

code three- to seven-character alphanumeric representation of a disease or condition

coexisting condition (comorbidity) additional illness that either has an effect on the patient's primary illness or is also treated during the encounter

combination code single code describing both the etiology and the manifestation(s) of a particular condition

convention typographic technique that provides visual guidance for understanding information

default code ICD-10-CM code listed next to the main term in the Alphabetic Index that is most often associated with a particular disease or condition

diagnostic statement physician's description of the main reason for a patient's encounter

eponym name or phrase formed from or based on a person's name

etiology cause or origin of a disease or condition

excludes 1 exclusion note used when two conditions could not exist together, such as an acquired and a congenital condition; means "not coded here"

excludes 2 exclusion note meaning that a particular condition is not included here, but a patient could have both conditions at the same time

exclusion note Tabular List entry limiting applicability of particular codes to specified conditions

external cause code ICD-10-CM code for an external cause of a disease or injury

first-listed code code for diagnosis that is the patient's main condition; in cases involving an underlying condition and a manifestation, the underlying condition is the first-listed code

GEM acronym for general equivalence mappings, reference tables of related ICD-10-CM and ICD-9-CM codes

ICD-10-CM HIPAA-mandated diagnosis code set as of October 1, 2015

ICD-10-CM Official Guidelines for Coding and Reporting general rules, inpatient (hospital) coding guidance, and outpatient (physician office/clinic) coding guidance from the four cooperating parties (CMS advisers and participants from the AHA, AHIMA, and NCHS)

inclusion note Tabular List entry addressing the applicability of certain codes to specified conditions

Index to External Causes index of all the external causes of diseases and injuries classified in the Tabular List

laterality use of ICD-10-CM classification system to capture the side of the body that is documented; the fourth, fifth, or sixth characters of a code specify the affected side(s)

main term word that identifies a disease or condition in the Alphabetic Index

manifestation a disease's typical signs, symptoms, or secondary processes

NEC (not elsewhere classified) abbreviation indicating the code to use when a disease or condition cannot be placed in any other category

Neoplasm Table summary table of code numbers for neoplasms by anatomical site and divided by the description of the neoplasm

nonessential modifier supplementary word or phrase that helps define a code in ICD-10-CM

NOS (not otherwise specified) indicates the code to use when no information is available for assigning the disease or condition a more specific code; unspecified

placeholder character (X) character "X" inserted in a code to fill a blank space

primary diagnosis first-listed diagnosis

principal diagnosis in inpatient coding, the condition established after study to be chiefly responsible for the admission of the patient

sequelae conditions that remain after an acute illness or injury has been treated and resolved

seventh-character extension necessary assignment of a seventh character to a code; often for the sequence of an encounter

subcategory four- or five-character code number

subterm word or phrase that describes a main term in the Alphabetic Index

Table of Drugs and Chemicals index in table format of drugs and chemicals that are listed in the Tabular List

Tabular List part of ICD-10-CM listing diagnosis codes in chapters alphanumerically

Z code abbreviation for codes from the twentieth chapter of ICD-10-CM that identify factors that influence health status and encounters that are not due to illness or injury

Medical Terminology: Reviewing Word Elements

Knowledge of medical terminology is required for coding diagnoses. Medical terms are made up of root words, prefixes, suffixes, and combining vowels and forms. The exercises here provide review of and practice with some key elements needed to correctly interpret medical documentation and then use the Alphabetic Index of ICD-10-CM to locate the main term(s).

Define the following word elements.

1. uter/o _____

2. cyst/o _____

3. phleb/o _____

4. gastro/ _____

5. hepat/o _____

6. encephal/o _____

7. osteo/o _____

8. hem/o, hemat/o _____

9. nephr/o _____

10. my/o _____

11. neur/o _____

12. dermato/o _____

13. myel/o _____

14. enter/o _____

15. col/o _____

16. cardi/o _____

17. arteri/o _____

18. arthr/o _____

19. cutane/o _____

20. esophag/o _____

Define the following prefixes and suffixes.

21. adeno– _____

22. –megaly _____

23. –esis _____

24. arterio– _____

25. chole– _____

26. melan– _____

27. –pathy _____

28. –itis _____

29. –phagia _____

30. dys– _____

31. brady– _____

32. ante– _____

33. hemi– _____

34. –cele _____

35. –algia _____

36. tachy– _____

37. –ectomy _____

38. –lysis _____

39. –plegia _____

40. –scopy _____

Factors Influencing Health Status and Contact with Health Services

Chapter 21: Codes Z00–Z99

Z codes, which make up Chapter 21 of ICD-10-CM, identify encounters for reasons other than illness or injury. Z codes are used for four main types of encounters: (1) healthy patients who receive services other than treatments, such as annual checkups, immunizations, and normal childbirth; (2) patients with known conditions for which they are receiving chemotherapy, radiation therapy, and rehabilitation aftercare; (3) patients with a problem that is not currently affecting their health status but that should be noted, such as a family history of a disease; and (4) patients being evaluated before an operation.

CODING TIP

Z Codes—Primary or Supplementary

Z codes are used as the primary code—that is, listed first—when healthy patients receive services, patients receive treatment for a current or resolving condition, and patients are evaluated preoperatively. Some Z codes, however, are never primary. Rather, these codes are always supplementary—they are additional codes that are listed after a primary code for the encounter.

A problem influencing a patient's health status that is not currently an illness or injury—such as a family history of a chronic disease—is an example of a supplementary Z code. In this case, the patient's reason for the encounter is listed first, followed by a Z code for the influencing factor.

Provide the Z code.

1. routine adult medical examination with no abnormal findings _____

2. exposure to tuberculosis _____

3. glaucoma screening _____

4. patient is a genetic carrier of cystic fibrosis _____

5. measles vaccination _____

6. admission for prophylactic removal of ovary _____

7. BMI of 46.9 in an adult patient _____

8. heart transplant (status post) _____

9. reinsertion of implantable subdermal contraceptive _____

10. contact with *E. coli* _____

Provide the Z code, and indicate whether it is a primary or a supplemental code.

11. preoperative cardiovascular examination _____

12. encounter for prophylactic rabies immune globin _____

13. observation of newborn for suspected infectious condition ruled out _____

14. counseling for tobacco abuse _____

15. supervision of normal first pregnancy _____

16. patient's parents are both deaf _____

17. history of allergy to latex _____

18. patient with hormone sensitive malignancy status _____

19. infection with penicillin-resistant microorganism _____

20. encounter for suture removal _____

Select the Z code for the following case studies.

21. A 55-year-old patient is new to the internist and presents today for his annual physical. During the discussion regarding the patient's medical history, he mentions that his father and grandfather had polycystic kidney disease, and he has some concerns regarding his potential for developing the same problem. In addition to the diagnosis code for the annual physical, what other diagnosis code would be needed? _____

22. A 35-year-old pregnant patient has asked her obstetrician to perform an amniocentesis. She has no specific anomalies or genetic predispositions, but is concerned for the well-being of her baby. No specific condition was found during the amniocentesis. What diagnosis code is used for the amniocentesis? _____

23. After a serious accident 2 months ago, a patient's left eye was removed. The patient now returns for fitting of the artificial eye that will replace the eye that was removed. _____

24. After testing of his patient's sister, the nephrologist determines that the sister is an appropriate candidate to donate a kidney for her brother's kidney transplant. Today, she is admitted to the hospital as a kidney donor. What diagnosis code is used for her hospital admission? _____

25. The patient has been seen by her gynecologist for close to 20 years, for her 3 pregnancies and a one-time abnormal pap smear. Today she is being seen for her annual routine pelvic exam. Which Z code is appropriate?

_____

NAME _____

External Causes of Morbidity

Chapter 20: Codes V00–Y99

External cause codes classify injuries resulting from environmental events such as falls, fires, and transportation accidents. The Alphabetic Index to External Causes that follows the Table of Drugs and Chemicals lists main terms for external causes—the accident, circumstance, or event that caused the injury.

CODING TIPS

External Cause Codes—A Supplementary Classification

External causes are not the primary diagnoses of patients' conditions, so these codes are never used alone. Instead, they always supplement a code that identifies the injury or condition itself. The primary diagnosis code is listed first, followed by the additional external cause code. Codes may be added to the first external cause code for the place of occurrence, activity, or status.

Seventh-Character Extensions

Many external cause codes for accidents and injuries require an extension as the seventh character for the visit sequence, if it is documented. The character A stands for the initial encounter; D for a subsequent encounter for this cause; and S for an encounter due to the sequela for this cause. Placeholder characters (X) may be needed to fill the spaces between a three-, four-, or five-character code and the seventh-character extension.

Provide the external cause codes for the following descriptions.

1. initial visit for fall from snowboard _____

2. motorcycle passenger injured in collision with bus in traffic accident,

   subsequent visit _____

3. patient suffered overexposure to radiation during therapy _____

4. hernia repair operation performed on the wrong patient _____

5. blood alcohol level of 60–79 mg/100 ml _____

6. accidental drowning in a lake _____

7. overexertion from repetitive movements, initial encounter _____

8. visit for treatment of residual effects of sunstroke _____

9. emergency room visit, jogger slipped on icy sidewalk _____

10. injury to driver in automobile collision with a cow _____

11. deep paper cut caused by an envelope _____

12. burn caused by flames from a fireplace _____

13. railway passenger injured while boarding the train _____

14. volunteer activity _____

15. accident due to text messaging while driving _____

Provide both the primary code for the patient's diagnosis and the external cause code in the correct order.

16. follow-up visit for fractured right elbow from fall when in-line roller skating _____

17. fractured thumb on right hand resulting from a fall from a ladder _____

18. contusions on left hand due to contact with a thorny cactus plant _____

19. patient tackled and knocked down during football game, suffers concussion with loss of consciousness for 20 minutes _____

20. driver's car was rear-ended by another car; patient has a spiral fracture of the left radius shaft _____

Select the external cause code(s) for the following case studies.

21. A patient was brought to the emergency department by ambulance after suffering a fractured left arm and left leg, with multiple soft tissue injuries. It was determined that the patient was the pilot of a commercial, fixed-wing, airplane flight that had crashed during a forced landing. _____

22. A patient was found unconscious at home after falling on the stairs to the second floor of her home. _____

23. A college student is brought to the emergency department after reportedly playing a blackout game with his friends. _____

24. An active-duty Army first sergeant was injured in Afghanistan when a gas bomb exploded during a night search of suspected enemy housing. _____

25. A patient was seen in the emergency department for pain in his right arm after accidentally falling off his bicycle. The emergency department physician determined the patient had injured the arm as a result of the bicycle fall. _____

Certain Infectious and Parasitic Diseases

Chapter 1: Codes A00–B99

Codes in this chapter classify communicable infectious and parasitic diseases. Most categories describe a condition and the type of organism that causes it. For example, category A03, shigellosis, describes acute infectious dysentery caused by *Shigella* bacteria. This category's codes classify four groups of bacteria plus a code for other *specified Shigella* infections, which occur infrequently, and a code for *unspecified* shigellosis for use when the condition is insufficiently described in the medical documentation for specific code assignment.

CODING TIP

"Includes" Notes

In the Tabular List, the word *includes* followed by descriptions of conditions helps the coder confirm the correct classification. These notes apply to the chapter, section, or category under which they appear. For example, the note *"Includes infection or foodborne intoxication due to any Salmonella species other than S. typhi and S. paratyphi"* appears beneath category A02, Other salmonella infections, and applies to infection or food poisoning caused by any organism in the category—that is, all the codes that begin with A02.

Provide the codes for the following diagnoses.

1. trichinosis _____

2. fever from Zika virus _____

3. Lyme disease _____

4. tabes dorsalis _____

5. ECHO virus _____

6. ovale malaria _____

7. Behçet's syndrome _____

8. primary genital syphilis _____

9. viral hepatitis A without mention of hepatic coma _____

10. rabies _____

11. tuberculous laryngitis, bacteriological examination not done _____

For the following descriptions, check the "Include" note when assigning the code.

12. acute hepatitis E without mention of hepatic coma _____

13. Malta fever _____

14. amebic skin ulceration due to *Entamoeba histolytica* _____

15. chronic gonococcal cystitis _____

16. recurrent tick-borne fever _____

17. pertussis due to *Bordetella bronchiseptica* _____

18. gonococcal endometritis, three months' duration _____

19. intestinal infection due to *Campylobacter* _____

20. shingles _____

Provide the codes for the following case studies.

21. A patient who had been exposed to AIDS (acquired immune deficiency syndrome) in the past developed symptoms of the disease, was tested, and learned that the results were positive for AIDS.

   _____

22. For weeks a patient was ill with diarrhea and abdominal pain. After examination and blood tests were completed, it was determined the patient suffered from enteritis caused by the astrovirus.

   _____

23. A patient was suffering from a yeast infection of the skin and finger-nails. She made an appointment with her physician, and after examination and blood work, he determined that she suffered from candidal onychia.

   _____

24. After 3 weeks of fever and chest pain, a patient was seen by his physician who determined that something was wrong with the patient's peri-cardium, the outer lining of the heart. After laboratory workup and testing, it was determined the patient had Coxsackie pericarditis.

   _____

25. A young patient with strep throat went untreated for over 3 weeks and developed scarlatina anginosa.

   _____

Neoplasms

Chapter 2: Codes C00–D49

Codes in this chapter of ICD-10-CM classify neoplasms, or tumors, which are growths that arise from normal tissue. Tumors are described according to their behavior as being one of four types: malignant (fast growing), benign (not spreading), of uncertain behavior (requiring further study), and of unspecified nature (insufficiently described for specific code assignment). Malignant tumors include primary, a tumor at the original site; secondary, a tumor that has spread, or *metastasized,* to another location from its primary site; and in situ, a noninvasive malignant tumor. Carcinoma in situ may also be referred to as *preinvasive cancer.*

In coding physicians' encounters with patients (outpatient coding), reporting suspected or possible conditions is avoided. Before pathology work identifies the behavior of a tumor, the condition can be classified with a code in the range R00–R99 (Symptoms, Signs and Abnormal Clinical and Laboratory Findings, Not Elsewhere Classified), if applicable, or from category Z12 (encounter for screening for malignant neoplasms).

CODING TIPS

The Neoplasm Table

The Alphabetic Index contains a Neoplasm Table that points to codes for neoplasms. The table lists the anatomical location in the first column. The next six columns classify the behavior of the neoplasm.

Multiple Lymph Node Sites

When coding lymph node neoplasms, if lymph nodes in more than one region of the body are involved, assign a code for multiple sites rather than codes for each site.

Using the Neoplasm Table in the Alphabetic Index, assign codes to the following diagnoses.

1. malignant primary neoplasm of the lower jawbone _____

2. benign neoplasm of the pharynx _____

3. neoplasm in situ, Wirsung's duct _____

4. neoplastic growth on the skin of the hip, uncertain behavior _____

   _____

5. secondary neoplasm on the posterior wall of the stomach _____

6. unspecified neoplasm of the pericardium _____

7. neoplasm of the mesopharynx, primary _____

8. cancer in situ, distal esophagus _____

9. benign tumor of the midbrain _____

10. spinal column neoplasm, primary _____

Using the Alphabetic Index and the Tabular List, provide codes for the following diagnoses.

11. unspecified, malignant carcinoid tumor of the hindgut _____

12. Hodgkin's granuloma, multiple lymph nodes _____

13. uterine fibromyoma _____

14. gastrointestinal stromal tumor of the jejunum _____

15. suspected primary carcinoma of the skin, screening test _____

16. ascites; possible carcinoma of the pancreas _____

17. cancer that has metastasized to the nose _____

18. Hodgkin's nodular sclerosis of the spleen _____

19. personal history of malignant neoplasm of the stomach _____

20. screening mammogram, patient has family history of breast cancer and is considered high risk *(two codes)* _____

Provide the codes for the following case studies.

21. After noticing a smallish dark irregular spot on her lip, the patient was seen by her internist who biopsied the site. The pathology report came back as malignant melanoma of the external lower lip. _____

22. While examining her patient during an annual physical, a physician noticed a nodule on the left shoulder. It was approximately 1 cm, and the physician was almost certain it was benign. She excised the nodule, and it was sent for pathology. The report indicated a dermatofibroma of the skin on the shoulder. _____

23. A patient with a history of abnormal pap smears is tested again. This time the result indicates a CINIII finding, or an in situ neoplasm of the cervix uteri. _____

24. This patient has a long history of respiratory infections, productive cough, and asthma. The physician has done recent testing to determine the cause of this extensive respiratory difficulty. The CT scan shows an anomaly, and the physician asks the patient to come in for another examination. His findings in the documentation indicate a neoplasm of the respiratory system. _____

25. Patient was in pain for several weeks in the sinus area. After ruling out sinusitis, the patient was referred to an otolaryngologist who examined the patient endoscopically and determined there was a lesion in the accessory sinuses. The lesion was biopsied, and the pathology report stated that the lesion was a carcinoma in situ of the accessory sinuses.

_____

Diseases of the Blood and Blood-Forming Organs and Certain Disorders Involving the Immune Mechanism

Chapter 3: Codes D50–D89

Codes in this chapter of ICD-10-CM classify diseases of the blood and blood-forming organs, such as anemia and coagulation defects. The chapter also covers disorders of the immune mechanism, such as graft-versus-host disease.

CODING TIP

"Excludes" Notes

In the Tabular List, the word *excludes* followed by descriptions of conditions helps the coder confirm a correct choice. Like *includes* notes, these guidelines can apply to the chapter, section, or category under which they appear. For example, in Chapter 3, a number of conditions are excluded from the entire chapter classification. Review the *Excludes 2* note to see the list of conditions that are not included in this chapter, such as autoimmune disease and HIV.

Provide the codes for the following diagnoses.

1. chlorotic anemia _____

2. vegan anemia due to dietary deficiency of vitamin B_{12} _____

3. sickle-cell anemia _____

4. hemophilia _____

5. hereditary hemolytic anemia _____

6. hereditary hemolytic anemia due to enzyme deficiency _____

7. monoclonal mast cell activation syndrome _____

8. specified hereditary hemolytic anemia not elsewhere classified _____

9. congenital elliptocytosis _____

10. iron deficiency anemia _____

11. Henoch's purpura _____

12. transient acquired pure red cell aplasia _____

13. hereditary sideroblastic anemia _____

14. congenital dyserythropoietic anemia _____

15. postprocedural hemorrhage of the spleen following a splenorrhaphy _____

Provide the codes for the following case studies.

16. After the birth of her first child, the patient bled profusely to the point of endangering her life. She mentioned to the obstetrician that her mother had had a similar problem when she was born. The lab results showed a deficiency in blood factor VII, indicative of von Willebrand's disease, which is congenital.

    _____

    _____

17. On several occasions, this patient noticed increased bleeding from even minor cuts or abrasions. Finally deciding to see her physician, the patient had lab work done, and the result indicated a low platelet count, with a diagnosis of thrombocytopenia.

    _____

    _____

18. After open heart surgery for blocked coronary arteries, the patient developed purplish spots on the leg that was used to harvest his vein for the graft material to be used in the heart bypass procedure. He had not injured the leg, but after years of smoking, his vascular system was compromised. After blood work was done, a diagnosis of secondary thrombocytopenia was given.

    _____

    _____

19. After years of untreated hypertension and development of end stage renal disease (ESRD), a patient also develops anemia. The physician explains that this is not an uncommon result of ESRD and gives an additional diagnosis of anemia in end stage renal disease.

    _____

    _____

20. A patient with fatigue, shortness of breath, and weakness is seen. Lab work indicates a deficiency in the red blood cell membrane, and a diagnosis of congenital nonspherocytic anemia, type II, is made.

    _____

    _____

Endocrine, Nutritional and Metabolic Diseases

Chapter 4: Codes E00–E89

Codes in this chapter of ICD-10-CM classify a variety of conditions. The most common disease is diabetes mellitus, which may be either type 1 or type 2. Another common condition is obesity, in which body weight is beyond skeletal and physical requirements because of excessive accumulation of body fat.

CODING TIPS

Coding for Diabetes Mellitus

Codes for diabetes mellitus combine (1) the type of diabetes mellitus, (2) what body system is affected, and (3) what complications also affect that body system. Most conditions can be described with a single code. For example, category code E11 indicates a diagnosis of type 2 diabetes mellitus. Under this category, the subcategories provide information about the related conditions, such as:

E11.0 Type 2 diabetes mellitus with hyperosmolarity

E11.2 Type 2 diabetes mellitus with kidney complications

E11.3 Type 2 diabetes mellitus with ophthalmic complications

E11.4 Type 2 diabetes mellitus with neurological complications

E11.5 Type 2 diabetes mellitus with circulatory complications

E11.6 Type 2 diabetes mellitus with other specified complications

Either a fifth, sixth, or seventh character, depending on the medical record, is required, such as:

E11.610 Type 2 diabetes mellitus with diabetic neuropathic arthropathy

More than one of these combination codes should be used to report all the conditions the patient has. If the type of diabetes (1 or 2) is not documented, the coder selects the appropriate choice from category E11, type 2 diabetes mellitus. The five diabetes mellitus categories are:

- E08 diabetes mellitus due to underlying condition
- E09 drug or chemical induced diabetes mellitus
- E10 type 1 diabetes mellitus
- E11 type 2 diabetes mellitus
- E13 other specified diabetes mellitus

Codes under category E08, diabetes mellitus due to underlying condition, and category E09, drug or chemical induced diabetes mellitus, indicate complications or manifestations that are associated with secondary diabetes mellitus. *Secondary* diabetes is always caused by some other condition or event, such as a malignant neoplasm of the pancreas or adverse effect from a drug. Whether to list secondary diabetes codes first or second is covered in the Tabular List instructions.

If the patient is insulin dependent, that is, routinely uses insulin, assign code Z79.4 as well.

Coding for Overweight and Obesity

Codes under category E66 are used to report the conditions of overweight and obese patients when documented. Fifth digits are assigned based on the cause of the condition, such as excess calories or drug-induced obesity.

For codes in category E66, an additional code should be assigned to identify body mass index (BMI), if known. These codes are located in the Z code chapter. Codes are available for adults (age 21 years or older) and for pediatric patients (age 2–20 years). These are the options for adults:

Z68.1 Body mass index (BMI) 19 or less, adult

Z68.2 Body mass index (BMI) 20–29, adult

    Z68.20 BMI 20.0–20.9, adult
    Z68.21 BMI 21.0–21.9, adult
    Z68.22 BMI 22.0–22.9, adult
    Z68.23 BMI 23.0–23.9, adult
    Z68.24 BMI 24.0–24.9, adult
    Z68.25 BMI 25.0–25.9, adult
    Z68.26 BMI 26.0–26.9, adult
    Z68.27 BMI 27.0–27.9, adult
    Z68.28 BMI 28.0–28.9, adult
    Z68.29 BMI 29.0–29.9, adult

Z68.3 Body mass index (BMI) 30–39, adult

    Z68.30 BMI 30.0–30.9, adult
    Z68.31 BMI 31.0–31.9, adult
    Z68.32 BMI 32.0–32.9, adult
    Z68.33 BMI 33.0–33.9, adult
    Z68.34 BMI 34.0–34.9, adult
    Z68.35 BMI 35.0–35.9, adult
    Z68.36 BMI 36.0–36.9, adult
    Z68.37 BMI 37.0–37.9, adult
    Z68.38 BMI 38.0–38.9, adult
    Z68.39 BMI 39.0–39.9, adult

Z68.4 Body mass index (BMI) 40 or greater, adult

    Z68.41 BMI 40.0–44.9, adult
    Z68.42 BMI 45.0–49.9, adult
    Z68.43 BMI 50.0–59.9, adult
    Z68.44 BMI 60.0–69.9, adult
    Z68.45 BMI 70.0 or greater, adult

Provide the codes for the following diagnoses.

1. congenital hypothyroidism _____

2. mucopolysaccharidosis _____

3. Zellweger syndrome _____

4. postsurgical hematoma of the thyroid following neck surgery _____

5. deficiency of vitamin K _____

6. medulloadrenal hyperfunction _____

7. kwashiorkor _____

8. familial hypercholesterolemia _____

9. Werner's syndrome _____

10. Lorain-Levi dwarfism _____

Note the fifth-, sixth-, or seventh-digit subclassification requirement when assigning codes for the following diagnoses.

11. Grave's disease _____

12. diabetes mellitus, type 1, with hyperglycemia _____

13. diabetes mellitus, type 2, without complications _____

14. diabetes with hypoglycemia, no coma _____

15. type 1 diabetes mellitus with Kimmelstiel-Wilson disease _____

16. type 2 diabetes mellitus with nonproliferative retinopathy with macular

    edema _____

17. goiter _____

18. morbid obesity in adult with BMI of 41 *(two codes)* _____

19. diabetes mellitus due to underlying condition with diabetic neuralgia

    _____

20. obese patient encounter for dietary counseling *(two codes)* _____

Provide the codes for the following case studies.

21. An adolescent boy has been seen annually by his internist who noticed a disturbing weight gain, some behavioral problems, and high blood sugar. Realizing the implication of this combination of problems could be based in the pituitary gland, the physician ordered tests and confirmed the diagnosis of Frohlich's syndrome. _____

22. Due to evidence of other metabolic disorders, a patient was asked to come in for urinalysis. The test results confirmed the physician's suspicion that amino acids were being excreted via the urine in abnormal amounts. The patient was diagnosed with cystinuria. _____

23. Patient presents with a 5-day history of excessive diarrhea and vomiting which has now resolved, but the patient is still unable to drink water or eat.

The physician suspects gastroenteritis and schedules the patient for testing. At this point, however, the physician indicates a diagnosis of dehydration. _____

24. Treating a 60-year-old patient, the physician notices a swelling in the neck area and determines that the patient's thyroid is enlarged on one side. After blood work, which indicates increased levels of the thyroid hormone, the physician diagnosed an acquired iodine-deficiency hypothyroidism. _____

25. A physician has been following a patient who recently arrived from a foreign country. As a result of his patient's depression, diarrhea, and unusual dermatitis, the physician orders lab work to determine what is the cause of his patient's symptoms. The result shows a niacin deficiency. On the basis of this finding, and the fact that the dermatitis is located only in body areas exposed to light, a diagnosis of pellagra is made. _____

Mental, Behavorial and Neurodevelopmental Disorders

Chapter 5: Codes F01–F99

Codes in this chapter of ICD-10-CM classify the various types of mental disorders, including conditions of drug and alcohol dependency, Alzheimer's disease, schizophrenic disorders, and mood disturbances.

CODING TIP

The Abbreviations NEC and NOS

NEC and NOS have different meanings and uses. NEC stands for not elsewhere classified. This abbreviation appears with a term when there is no code that is specific for the condition. It means that no code matches the particular problem described in the diagnostic statement. In this case, the coder has specific documentation, but ICD-10-CM does not provide a code that matches the statement. NOS, which stands for not otherwise specified, means that the diagnostic statement does not provide enough information to classify the condition.

Provide the codes for the following diagnoses.

1. mild mental retardation _____

2. premenstrual dysphoric disorder _____

3. frontal lobe syndrome _____

4. tobacco dependence _____

5. subacute delirium _____

6. nonalcoholic Korsakoff's psychosis _____

7. neurotic anxiety disorder _____

8. depression with anxiety _____

9. panic attack _____

10. hoarding disorder _____

11. episodic cocaine abuse _____

12. compulsive neurosis _____

13. severe mixed manic-depressive psychosis _____

14. chronic catatonic-type schizophrenic disorder _____

15. occasional amphetamine abuse _____

16. adolescent gender dysphoria _____

17. dependence on barbiturates and morphine _____

Provide the codes for the following case studies.

18. The patient presents with a 10-year history of drug abuse and is being seen today for evaluation of a 2-year history of continuous dependence on methadone.

    _____

    _____

19. Due to complaints from the school, a pediatrician is examining a 5-year-old child who is having mild tantrums so often that his parents are concerned that there is something physically wrong with him. The school feels the tantrums go beyond what is expected for the child's age. No physical explanation is found on examination.

    _____

    _____

20. A patient was brought to the emergency room after hours of rapid, excited speech, unexplained laughter, and constant, rapid movements. Friends were unable to determine why this was happening and were concerned. No drugs were found, and the physician decided this was a single episode of manic disorder and recommended the patient see his own physician the next day for a complete workup.

    _____

    _____

Diseases of the Nervous System
Diseases of the Eye and Adnexa
Diseases of the Ear and Mastoid Process

Chapter 6: Codes G00–G99

Chapter 7: Codes H00–H59

Chapter 8: Codes H60–H95

Codes in these chapters of ICD-10-CM classify diseases of the central nervous system, the peripheral nervous system, the eye, and the ear.

CODING TIP

"Code First Underlying Disease" Instruction

Some conditions require the assignment of two codes, one for the disease's etiology (origin or cause) and a second for its manifestation, or typical signs or symptoms. (On the other hand, it is common in ICD-10-CM to assign combination codes for conditions due to certain causes.) In the Alphabetic Index, a requirement for two codes is indicated when two codes appear after a term, the second of which is in brackets. Likewise, the instruction "code first underlying disease" in the Tabular List indicates the need for two codes. (The alternative phrases "code first associated disorder" or "code first underlying disorder" may also be used.) The instruction appears below a code needing two codes. Codes shown in italics are never primary. These codes are for the *manifestation* only, not for the etiology, even when the diagnostic statement is written in that order.

Provide the codes for the following diagnoses.

1. Huntington's chorea _____

2. hereditary spastic paraplegia _____

3. paralysis _____

4. bilateral femoral nerve lesions _____

5. benign intracranial hypertension _____

6. blindness in right eye; low vision in left eye _____

7. cortical senile cataract _____

8. causalgia of both arms _____

9. visual field defect _____

10. tributary retinal vein occlusion of the right eye with macular edema _____

Provide either etiology and manifestation codes in the correct order or a combination code, as required. *Hint:* **Remember to check for seventh-character extension requirements.**

11. toxic encephalitis due to undetermined exposure to mercury _____

12. childhood cerebral degeneration due to Hunter's disease _____

13. peripheral autonomic neuropathy due to metabolic disease _____

14. Lambert-Eaton syndrome due to malignant neoplasm of left main

    bronchus _____

15. myopathy from Addison's disease _____

16. retinal dystrophy due to a lipid storage disorder _____

17. early-onset cerebellar ataxia with retained tendon reflexes _____

18. diabetic cataract _____

19. exophthalmic ophthalmoplegia due to toxic diffuse goiter _____

20. chronic mycotic otitis externa right because of otomycosis _____

Provide the codes for the following case studies.

21. Patient presents today with difficulty in producing tears. After examination the physician determined that the tear sac, or lacrimal sac, was narrowed. The diagnosis is stenosis of the lacrimal sac. _____

22. After suffering for 3 days with a fever and ear pain, the patient was seen by her physician. Upon examination the physician diagnosed an acute case of serous otitis media. _____

23. A patient with both chronic and acute sinusitis comes in today because of a constant ringing in her right ear. Upon examination the physician determines that she has subjective tinnitus because the sound can only be heard by the patient. _____

24. After 2 days of discharge and redness in both eyes, a patient is seen by his internist. The internist determined the patient was suffering from conjunctivitis, specifically mucopurulent conjunctivitis. _____

25. Patient notices a halo around street lights and traffic lights when driving at night. She has also noticed a lessening in her peripheral vision. Her ophthalmologist examines her eyes with the ophthalmoscope and does visual field testing. The results of these examinations indicate bilateral, moderate-stage, primary open-angle glaucoma. _____

Diseases of the Circulatory System

Chapter 9: Codes I00–I99

Codes in this chapter of ICD-10-CM classify a large group of circulatory system disorders. Many are complex, involving heart disease and serious vascular disorders.

CODING TIP

Ischemic Heart Disease

Ischemic heart disease conditions—those caused by reduced blood flow to the heart—are coded under categories I20–I25. Myocardial infarctions that are acute or have a documented duration of four weeks (28 days) or less are located in category I21. Subsequent myocardial infarctions occurring within four weeks (28 days) of a previous acute MI are assigned to category I22. A code from category I22 is used along with a code from category I21. Once the MI has gone past four weeks (28 days) in duration without current symptoms, it is considered an *old myocardial infarction* and is coded to I25.2. Other chronic ischemic heart diseases are coded under category I25. An unspecified acute MI is coded to the default I21.3. Note that the MI, subsequent MI, and chronic ischemic heart disease require additional codes, when applicable, to report environmental factors such as history of tobacco use.

Provide the codes for the following diagnoses.

1. acute rheumatic endocarditis _____

2. chronic rheumatic pericarditis _____

3. unstable angina pectoris _____

4. cerebral infarction to thrombosis of bilateral posterior arteries _____

5. atherosclerosis of nonautologous biological coronary bypass grafts with

   unstable angina pectoris _____

6. primary pulmonary hypertension _____

7. acute endocarditis _____

8. constrictive pericarditis _____

9. postprocedural hypotension _____

10. vertebral artery aneurysm _____

11. heart failure following cardiac surgery _____

12. meningococcal infective endocarditis _____

13. Spens' syndrome _____

14. acute myocardial infarction 8 weeks ago _____

15. initial care of acute ST elevation myocardial infarction of anterolateral
    wall _____

16. occlusion of basilar artery with cerebral infarction _____

17. cerebral thrombosis left posterior cerebral artery _____

18. stenosis of vertebral artery _____

19. Beck's syndrome _____

20. sick sinus _____

Provide the codes for the following case studies.

21. A 70-year-old man has been experiencing shortness of breath and fatigue.
    His internist referred him to a cardiologist who performed a stress test that
    was abnormal. An echocardiogram indicated a problem on the right side of
    the heart. A cardiac catheterization was performed, and it was determined
    that the patient suffered from rheumatic tricuspid valve obstruction.

    _____

22. Three years ago this patient suffered an acute myocardial infarction.
    He has been treated with medication, exercise, and diet; after 8 weeks his
    condition was no longer considered acute. He comes in today for his
    3-year follow-up visit, and he is completely without any symptoms.
    His diagnosis is healed (old) myocardial infarction.

    _____

23. A patient has been complaining of chest pain, but his EKGs and a stress
    test are normal. An echocardiogram is performed showing layers of the
    pericardium had adhered to each other. Diagnosis: Soldier's patches.

    _____

24. A patient with long-term liver disease has his blood work checked. Lab
    results indicate a low hematocrit, and his physician suspects internal
    bleeding. An esophagoscopy is done showing that the patient has bleeding
    esophageal varicose veins.

    _____

25. A patient calls his internist. He feels like he is suffocating and he has chest
    pain. It started when he was running with his grandchildren. He noticed a
    similar reaction after cutting the lawn recently. After examination, EKG,
    and an attempted stress test, the physician diagnosed stenocardia.

    _____

Diseases of the
Circulatory System *continued*

CODING TIP

Hypertension

Hypertension is a diagnosis related to high blood pressure. Almost all cases are due to unknown causes. This is called essential hypertension and is the primary diagnosis. Category I10 is used to code all the following: high blood pressure and arterial, benign, essential, malignant, primary, or systemic hypertension.

In some cases, the hypertension is due to an underlying condition; this is called secondary hypertension. A code from category I15 is listed after the etiology (cause) code.

Note that a diagnosis of hypertension is different from elevated blood-pressure reading. That finding, without a formal, specific diagnosis of hypertension, is coded to Chapter 18, Symptoms, Signs and Abnormal Clinical and Laboratory Findings, Not Elsewhere Classified, category R03.

Note that the hypertension categories require additional codes, when applicable, to report environmental factors such as history of tobacco use.

Using the hypertensive disease categories, assign codes to the following diagnoses.

26. benign hypertension due to brain tumor _____

27. unspecified hypertension due to renal artery stenosis _____

28. secondary malignant hypertension due to Cushing's disease _____

29. hypertensive urgency _____

30. intermittent vascular hypertensive disease _____

Following the normal procedure, provide the codes for the following diagnoses. Some diagnoses require multiple codes.

31. rheumatic aortic insufficiency and congestive heart failure _____

32. mitral and aortic valve insufficiency and persistent atrial flutter _____

33. acute pericarditis caused by chronic uremia _____

34. left heart failure due to benign hypertension _____

35. hematoma of the heart following cardiac bypass surgery _____

36. cardiomyopathy due to excessive alcohol consumption _____

37. angina pectoris and essential hypertension _____

38. calcified tuberculosis with endocarditis _____

39. peripheral angiopathy due to diabetes mellitus _____

40. memory deficiency after a nontraumatic subarachnoid hemorrhage _____

Diseases of the Respiratory System

Chapter 10: Codes J00–J99

Codes in this chapter of ICD-10-CM classify respiratory illnesses such as pneumonia, chronic obstructive pulmonary disease, and asthma.

CODING TIP

Chronic versus Acute Conditions

Acute conditions—those with relatively sudden or severe problems—are reported with the specific code that is designated acute, if provided in ICD-10-CM. Chronic conditions—those that continue over a long period of time or recur frequently—are reported each time the patient receives care for that condition. Some encounters cover treatment for both an acute and a chronic condition. If both an acute illness and a chronic condition are treated in an encounter and each has a code, list the acute code first. In some cases, a single code covers both types of the condition, so only one code is reported.

Provide the codes for the following diagnoses.

1. bronchiectasis without acute exacerbation _____

2. adenoid vegetations _____

3. deviated nasal septum _____

4. cellulitis of vocal cords _____

5. nasopharyngeal polyp _____

6. peritonsillar abscess _____

7. chronic mediastinitis _____

8. lung abscess _____

9. allergic bronchopulmonary aspergillosis _____

10. influenza due to identified novel influenza A virus _____

Some of the following diagnoses require two codes.

11. pneumonia in cytomegalic inclusion disease _____

12. pneumonia due to *Pseudomonas* _____

13. acute and chronic respiratory failure _____

14. adenoviral pneumonia and allergic bronchitis _____

15. asthma with chronic obstructive pulmonary disease _____

16. acute bronchitis with chronic obstructive pulmonary disease _____

17. acute pulmonary manifestations due to radiation _____

18. hematoma of the trachea following an unrelated procedure _____

19. hyperplasia of tonsils with adenoids _____

20. acute bronchiolitis due to RSV _____

Provide the codes for the following case studies.

21. After moving to South Carolina, a patient noticed increasing shortness of breath and wheezing, and was diagnosed with asthma. This morning she presents with greater difficulty in breathing and her wheezing has become much worse—it had started suddenly during the night.

_____

22. A 12-year-old boy starts complaining of itchy eyes, runny nose, sneezing; he says he feel stuffy. His problem seems to coincide with the trees and flowers starting to bloom. His pediatrician diagnosed allergic rhinitis from exposure to pollen.

_____

23. The patient presents with a 2-year history of a productive cough with unknown etiology, which is now more severe. The physician documents a diagnosis of acute and chronic obstructive bronchitis.

_____

24. After 2 weeks of throat pain, the patient realized that he also was running a fever. After dealing with the fever for 3 days, he sees his physician, who indicates a diagnosis of acute infective tonsillitis.

_____

25. A 32-year-old patient with virtually a lifetime history of allergies has been seeing her physician almost five times a year for pain in the area behind her cheekbones and purulent nasal discharge. The physician documents that the patient has chronic maxillary sinus infections.

_____

Diseases of the Digestive System

Chapter 11: Codes K00–K95

Codes in this chapter of ICD-10-CM classify diseases of the digestive system. Codes are listed according to anatomical location, beginning with the oral cavity and continuing through the intestines.

CODING TIP

Digestive System Combination Codes

Some digestive system conditions in ICD-10-CM are classified with combination codes that cover both the illness, such as gastric or peptic ulcers, and a commonly associated condition, such as hemorrhage (bleeding) and/or perforation. Check carefully during the coding process to verify whether a combination code classifies both the etiology and the manifestation of the documented diagnosis.

Provide the codes for the following diagnoses.

1. anal abscess _____

2. appendicitis _____

3. reflux esophagitis _____

4. impacted teeth _____

5. severe localized periodontitis _____

6. GERD with esophagitis _____

7. irritable bowel syndrome with constipation _____

8. irreversible pulpitis _____

9. sialoadenitis _____

10. perforated esophagus _____

11. toxic megacolon _____

12. fecal impaction _____

13. cholostatic cirrhosis _____

Some of the following diagnoses require two codes.

14. food protein-induced enterocolitis due to allergy to eggs _____

15. hepatitis in Coxsackie virus disease _____

16. gastrojejunal ulcer with obstruction, hemorrhage, and perforation

    _____

17. strawberry gallbladder _____

18. acute and chronic cholecystitis _____

19. recurrent bilateral inguinal hernia _____

20. liver damage because of chronic alcoholism _____

Provide the codes for the following case studies.

21. Patient complains of difficulty swallowing with an almost constant
    burning sensation in the lower chest area. An x-ray is performed with
    fluoroscopy. The x-ray shows a protrusion/hernia of the stomach through
    the opening of the esophagus where it joins the stomach (esophageal
    hiatus).

    _____

22. Two months after surgery for a partial colectomy, the patient comes in to
    see his surgeon for ongoing abdominal pain. Upon examination, the
    surgeon finds adhesions in the patient's peritoneum.

    _____

23. A dialysis patient who recently changed over to continual ambulatory
    peritoneal dialysis complains of abdominal pain. The physician determines
    that the patient has peritonitis.

    _____

24. A patient has been suffering with stomach pain, cramps, and diarrhea for
    2 months; her weight is dropping dramatically. The physician orders a
    CT scan, and the findings indicate Crohn's disease.

    _____

25. Patient has suffered for years with stomach pain and now sees his
    physician because he has started vomiting. In the course of their discus-
    sion the patient mentions that he gets some relief from drinking milk. The
    physician schedules an endoscopy and finds a perforated peptic ulcer.

    _____

Diseases of the Skin and Subcutaneous Tissue

Chapter 12: Codes L00–L99

Codes in this chapter of ICD-10-CM classify conditions such as acne, dermatitis, skin lesions, rosacea, melasma, abscesses, cellulitis, severe pressure ulcers, and ischemic ulcers.

CODING TIP

Pressure Ulcers

Pressure ulcers, category L89, are a common condition in many inpatient and long-term-care healthcare settings. Coding is based on selecting a combination code that reports both the site and the stage of the ulcer. The stage is reported with a sixth digit, as follows:

Unstageable (digit 0): stage cannot be determined due to some circumstance such as prior treatment with a skin flap or graft or coverage with scar tissue.

Stage 1 (digit 1): observable pressure-related alteration of intact skin.

Stage 2 (digit 2): partial-thickness skin loss involving epidermis, dermis, or both.

Stage 3 (digit 3): full-thickness skin loss involving damage to, or necrosis of, subcutaneous tissue that may extend down to, but not through, underlying fascia.

Stage 4 (digit 4): full-thickness skin loss with extensive destruction, tissue necrosis, or damage to muscle, bone, or supporting structures (such as tendon, joint, or capsule).

Unspecified stage (digit 9): documentation refers to a healing ulcer that does not have a specified stage.

Note that completely healed pressure ulcers are not coded.

Provide the codes for the following diagnoses.

1. allergic urticaria _____

2. sebaceous cyst _____

3. hirsutism _____

4. ingrowing nail _____

5. acquired keratoderma _____

6. clavus _____

7. lichenification _____

8. large plaque parapsoriasis _____

9. Ritter's disease _____

10. dermatosis herpetiformis _____

11. DSAP (disseminated superficial actinic porokeratosis) _____

12. herald patch (pityriasis rosea) _____

13. periorbital cellulitis _____

14. psoriatic arthropathy _____

15. third-degree sunburn _____

Provide a combination code correctly reflecting the pressure ulcer site and stage for the following diagnostic statements.

16. right ankle has a healing, stage 2 pressure ulcer _____

17. pressure ulcer on head not stageable due to prior treatment with skin graft

_____

18. pressure ulcer, healing, left heel _____

19. pressure ulcer, healing, stage 3, left hip _____

20. patient had pressure ulcer that has completely healed _____

Provide codes for the following case studies.

21. A teenage patient volunteers to help out at the local homeless shelter. She offers to do dishes there every day after school. After 2 weeks, she realizes that the rash she has developed is not going away, and she sees her doctor who recognizes that she has contact dermatitis caused by the dish detergent.

_____

22. An active, healthy 50-year-old patient is distressed to find several groups of skin eruptions on her lower abdomen and under her arms. Her internist sends her to a dermatologist who diagnoses Sneddon-Wilkinson syndrome.

_____

23. A middle-aged female patient has recently completed an intense, year-long diet, and has lost an extreme amount of weight. As a result of the lost weight, the patient has excessive loose skin around her torso.

_____

24. An elderly man is hospitalized and subsequently placed on a ventilator. Due to his condition he is unable to move on his own or to be moved. As a result, he develops a stage 1 decubitus ulcer on his left lower back.

_____

25. A young patient arrives 3 days after having a cyst excised. Due to this previous dermatological procedure, he now has a serious hematoma below his skin near the site of the operation.

_____

NAME _____

Diseases of the Musculoskeletal System and Connective Tissue

Chapter 13: Codes M00–M99

Codes in this chapter of ICD-10-CM classify conditions of the bones and joints—arthropathies (joint disorders), dorsopathies (back disorders), rheumatism, and other diseases.

CODING TIPS

Site and Laterality

Many of the thousands of codes in Chapter 13 are selected by *site*—the bone, joint, or muscle affected—and the *laterality*—left, right, or unspecified. Some conditions, such as osteoporosis, may affect more than one site, however, and under those categories codes are listed for multiple sites. If no multiple-site code is available, use as many single-site codes as needed to report the condition(s).

Pathological versus Traumatic Fractures

Pathological fractures, those due to bone illness, can affect patients with conditions such as bone metastasis, severe osteoporosis, or osteoarthritis. These fractures are coded from Chapter 13. If the fracture is due to trauma, a code from the pathologic fracture category is not assigned; the injury is coded from Chapter 19.

Provide the codes for the following diagnoses.

1. hallux varus, right great toe _____

2. senile osteoporosis _____

3. bunion _____

4. limb pain _____

5. pain in lower back _____

6. tailor's bunion on the left foot _____

7. Schmorl's nodes of the lumbar region _____

8. calcaneal spur _____

9. patellar chondromalacia _____

10. systemic sclerosis _____

11. old rupture of meniscus of scapula _____

12. right temporomandibular arthralgia _____

13. Paget's bone disease _____

14. aseptic necrosis of medial femoral condyle _____

15. C6–C7 cervical disc disorder with myelopathy _____

16. upper arm arthropathy in Behçet's syndrome _____

17. pericarditis in systemic lupus erythematosus _____

18. right shoulder osteopathy due to sequelae infantile paralytic poliomyelitis

    (two codes) _____

19. chronic multifocal osteomyelitis of glenohumeral joint and elbow joint

    _____

20. ruptured extensor and flexor tendons, hand (two codes) _____

Provide the codes for the following case studies.

21. The patient complains of pain in the right lower leg. No injury has occurred, and the patient is otherwise healthy. A CT scan reveals osteomyelitis of the lower leg, and her physician further specifies her condition as subacute.

    _____

22. A patient who received an internal prosthetic right hip 6 months ago recently suffered a fall and has returned for a second time since that fall with a report of continuing pain in her hip. At her previous visit, x-rays were taken, and the radiologist identified a traumatic periprosthetic fracture around the internal prosthetic right hip joint.

    _____

23. Five months ago, the patient suffered a pathological left ankle fracture. He is still in pain and feels that "something's not right." X-rays are taken of the original fracture site, and the findings are that the ankle has healed in misalignment—a malunion. (*Hint:* Remember the seventh-character extension for the subsequent visit for a malunion.)

    _____

24. A 7-year-old boy is brought to the doctor because his left foot has turned inward and the heel has raised up. The problem may be a result of the boy's cerebral palsy, but this problem would have appeared earlier. For now the physician indicates he has acquired club foot of the left leg.

    _____

25. A 12-year-old's parents notice that their daughter is walking differently and appears to favor one side. They bring her to the pediatrician who finds that the patient has a sideward curvature of the spine in the T1–T12 area, or thoracogenic scoliosis.

    _____

Diseases of the Genitourinary System

Chapter 14: Codes N00–N99

Codes in this chapter of ICD-10-CM classify diseases of the male and female genitourinary (GU) systems, such as infections of the genital tract, renal disease, conditions of the prostate, and problems with the cervix, vulva, and breast. Note that some components of this system, including the kidneys, ureters, and fallopian tubes, do not have codes for laterality.

CODING TIP

Chronic Kidney Disease (CKD)

Chronic kidney disease (CKD) is coded based on the documented stage, from stage 1 to 5, and a sixth level, end stage renal disease (ESRD), in which the patient needs dialysis chronically. If the cause of CKD is diabetes mellitus or hypertension, code sequence is based on Tabular List conventions.

Provide the codes for the following diagnoses.

1. renal failure _____

2. ureteric stone _____

3. mobile kidney _____

4. chronic interstitial cystitis _____

5. abscess of the breast and nipple _____

6. male infertility _____

7. pain in the scrotum _____

8. acute salpingitis and oophoritis _____

9. uterine endometriosis _____

10. fallopian tube torsion _____

Provide two codes for each of the following diagnostic statements. Remember to list codes in the correct order, if it is specified.

11. uremic pericarditis _____

12. prostatic hyperplasia with urge and stress incontinence _____

13. prostatitis in blastomycosis _____

14. acute vaginitis due to *Staphylococcus* _____

15. female infertility due to postoperative peritubal adhesions (three codes)

    _____

16. acute cystitis due to *Escherichia coli* organism _____

17. nephritis due to diabetes mellitus _____

18. pyelonephritis due to renal tuberculosis _____

19. acute prostatitis with hematuria due to *Streptococcus* _____

20. vulvovaginal gland abscess and female stress incontinence

    _____

Provide the codes for the following case studies.

21. The patient is seen for her annual gynecological exam, and a pap smear is taken. The results show a mild dysplasia of the cervix. _____

22. A 30-year-old woman has recently started doing her own breast exams and notices a bumpy consistency to her breasts, with some mild pain, particularly just before and after her menstrual period. Due to her concern, she sees her gynecologist who after examining her documents a diagnosis of fibrocystic breast disease of both breasts. _____

23. A 58-year-old woman sees her gynecologist because she is having urinary problems. She complains that when she sneezes or coughs, she urinates involuntarily, even though she has recently emptied her bladder. It even occurs when she tries to lift one of her grandchildren. The physician diagnoses stress incontinence. _____

24. A patient with a 6-year history of adult onset diabetes is seen for follow-up of her diabetic condition. The physician does lab work and weighs the patient who shows a considerable weight gain and edema. The lab work results indicate a large amount of protein in the urine. The physician documents nephrosis. _____

25. A 47-year-old man underwent successful interstitial seed therapy on his prostate 4 months ago. However, today he has arrived to report that he is having difficulty maintaining an erection. The physician documents erectile dysfunction following the interstitial seed therapy procedure.

    _____

Pregnancy, Childbirth and the Puerperium

Chapter 15: Codes O00–O9A

Codes in this chapter of ICD-10-CM classify conditions that are involved with pregnancy, childbirth, and the puerperium. Most codes require a final character for the trimester of pregnancy, whether the first (less than 14 weeks/0 days), the second (14 weeks to 28 weeks/0 days), or third (28 weeks/0 days until delivery).

CODING TIPS

Mothers' Conditions

Codes in this chapter (Chapter 15) of ICD-10-CM are assigned to conditions of the mother only, not of the infant. They cover the course of pregnancy and childbirth from conception through the puerperium, which is the 6-week period following delivery. Codes for conditions that affect newborns are in ICD-10-CM's Chapter 16.

Normal Pregnancy

Supervision of normal pregnancy, such as routine prenatal outpatient visit, is reported with a code from category Z34. The Z codes are not to be used along with the Chapter 15 codes for outpatient coding.

Provide the codes for the following diagnoses.

1. hydatidiform mole _____

2. abdominal pregnancy without intrauterine pregnancy _____

3. complete spontaneous abortion complicated by renal failure _____

4. incomplete spontaneous abortion with complications _____

5. legally induced abortion _____

6. complete abortion complicated by shock _____

7. maternal hypertension complicating childbirth _____

8. hemorrhage in early pregnancy _____

9. low-lying placenta with hemorrhage, second trimester _____

10. mild hyperemesis gravidarum _____

11. Rh incompatibility _____

12. delivery complicated by short umbilical cord _____

13. gestational edema complicating the puerperium _____

14. nipple fissure in fourth week after childbirth _____

15. delivery complicated by inverted uterus _____

16. postpartum fibrinolysis _____

Provide two codes for each of the following diagnostic statements. Remember to list codes in the correct order, if it is specified.

17. normal delivery of single liveborn _____

18. normal delivery of liveborn twins _____

19. normal delivery of quadruplets, three liveborn and one stillborn

_____

20. delivery complicated by obstructed labor caused by face presentation

_____

Provide the codes for the following case studies.

21. A pregnant patient presents shortly before delivering her second child but first requires maternal care due to a vertical scar from the cesarean delivery of her first child.

_____

22. The patient is frazzled to find herself still pregnant after 41 weeks. She had planned to deliver after the "normal" 39 weeks and is having difficulty adjusting to this delay.

_____

23. This 30-year-old is seeing her obstetrician during her first pregnancy for regular follow-up care during her 25th week of pregnancy. She mentions the swelling in her legs and unusual fatigue. The physician does a blood workup, which reveals an abnormal blood glucose. He reassures his patient that she does not have diabetes but what is referred to as gestational diabetes, and he fully expects her blood glucose to return to normal after the baby is delivered.

_____

24. A day after delivering her baby, the patient finds herself in additional discomfort and discovers a swollen area on her vulva. The obstetrician comes in to examine her and finds she has a hematoma.

_____

25. During the eighth month of her pregnancy, the patient contacts her obstetrician because of the discomfort from the baby's position. She is also experiencing a swollen, reddened area on her calf that is painful. The obstetrician has her come in immediately and finds she has a deep vein thrombosis on the left leg. The patient is informed she must get off her feet and lie with the leg elevated, using warm compresses.

_____

Certain Conditions Originating in the Perinatal Period

Chapter 16: Codes P00–P96

Codes in this chapter of ICD-10-CM classify conditions of the fetus or the newborn infant, the neonate, up to 28 days after birth.

CODING TIP

Infants' Conditions

Codes in this chapter of ICD-10-CM (Chapter 16) are assigned only to conditions of the infant, not of the mother. (Codes for conditions that affect the management of the mother's pregnancy are in Chapter 15.) They cover the perinatal period, which is the period from shortly before birth until 28 days following delivery. When the hospitalization that results in the birth is to be coded, these codes are secondary to codes from category Z38, Liveborn infants according to place of birth and type of delivery. Note that codes are available to report low birth weight and prematurity if documented.

Provide the codes for the following diagnoses.

1. newborn infant weighing 800 grams _____

2. newborn affected by mother's use of alcohol _____

3. newborn affected by the mother's malnutrition _____

4. small newborn weighing 2600 grams _____

5. respiratory distress syndrome in newborn _____

6. fever in newborn _____

7. anemia of prematurity _____

8. newborn affected by forceps delivery _____

9. neonatal superficial hematoma _____

10. congenital rubella _____

11. neonatal *Candida* infection _____

12. moderate birth asphyxia _____

Provide Z codes and codes from Chapter 16 for the following diagnoses.

13. hospital vaginal delivery of living child, infant is premature and weighs

2000 grams _____

14. hospital birth of twin, mate liveborn, neonatal pulmonary immaturity

_____

15. full-term birth in hospital of living male child, delivered by cesarean

section, with neonatal transient hyperthyroidism

_____

16. postterm birth in hospital of twin, mate stillborn (code for the surviving twin)

_____

17. birth at 36 completed weeks of immature female, delivered in ambulance

en route to hospital _____

Provide the codes for the following case studies.

18. Shortly after the birth episode had ended, the newborn was taking quick
breaths, indicating shallow breathing, with some evidence of cyanosis.
After her examination, the pediatrician reassured the parents it was a
transitory problem that would resolve on its own in about 3 days, but they
would give the baby some oxygen in the meantime—the condition is often
referred to as wet lung syndrome.

_____

_____

19. A pediatrician became concerned when he noticed that the newborn was
somewhat jaundiced and had an enlarged spleen, in addition to a light for
dates weight of only 2550 grams. Laboratory studies showed that the
newborn suffered from anemia caused by RH isoimmunization.

_____

_____

20. Shortly before her labor started, a patient became short of breath and had
difficulty walking. Her examination at the hospital showed an excess of
amniotic fluid or hydramnios, which would account for her symptoms.

_____

_____

Congenital Malformations, Deformations and Chromosomal Abnormalities

Chapter 17: Codes Q00–Q99

Codes in this brief ICD-10-CM chapter classify anomalies, malformations, and diseases that exist at birth. Unlike acquired disorders, congenital conditions are either hereditary or due to influencing factors during gestation.

CODING TIP

Congenital Anomalies and Patients' Ages

Although congenital anomalies are defined as existing at birth, they do not always immediately affect the patient. As examples, normal human beings have 33 vertebrae, but a person without the normal number may be asymptomatic, and patients with dominant polycystic disease may not experience impaired function until adulthood. The classifications for congenital anomalies thus are not related to patients' ages.

Provide the codes for the following diagnoses.

1. congenital absence of aplasia of aorta _____
2. unilateral congenital hip dislocation _____
3. left side longitudinal vaginal setpum with microperforate _____
4. undescended testis _____
5. congenital cystic liver disease _____
6. Hirschsprung's disease _____
7. arterial tortuosity syndrome _____
8. web of larynx _____
9. scimitar syndrome _____
10. posterior atresia of nares _____
11. cleft palate with cleft lip _____
12. annular pancreas _____
13. autosomal dominant polycystic kidney _____
14. bilateral fused toes _____

15. metatarsus adductus, congenital _____

16. translocation Down's syndrome _____

17. hereditary trophedema _____

Provide the codes for the following case studies.

18. A newborn has difficulty breathing almost immediately after birth. The pediatrician's examination shows that the larynx is narrowed, almost completely stenosed, and an alternative airway needs to be created immediately.

    _____

    _____

19. A newborn shows difficulty with urination. The examination reveals that the urethra has failed to develop, causing a urethral stricture (atresia).

    _____

    _____

20. Shortly after a baby's birth, the pediatrician finds a dilated bladder and ureters and the absence of the lower rectus abdominis muscle, also known as prune belly syndrome.

    _____

    _____

Symptoms, Signs and Abnormal Clinical and Laboratory Findings, Not Elsewhere Classified

Chapter 18: Codes R00–R99

Codes in this chapter of ICD-10-CM classify patients' symptoms, signs, abnormal results of clinical or other tests and procedures, and ill-defined conditions for which a definitive diagnosis cannot be made. In physician coding, these codes are always used instead of coding "rule out," "probable," or "suspected" conditions.

CODING TIPS

Combination Codes for Typical Symptoms

A number of combination codes identify both the diagnosis and its common symptoms. In these situations, additional codes for the symptoms are not reported.

HIV Codes

HIV coding is complex. When a diagnosis of HIV infection has been made, code B20 is used to classify any of the many terms used for this condition, such as AIDS (acquired immunodeficiency syndrome) and HIV disease. When a patient with no related symptoms has a screening test for HIV infection, code Z11.4 is used. If the test results are positive for HIV infection but the patient shows no symptoms, code Z21 is used. If, however, the test result is reported as "nonspecific (inconclusive) serologic evidence of HIV," code R75 is used.

Provide the codes for the following diagnoses.

1. coma _____

2. prediabetes _____

3. abnormal electrocardiogram _____

4. asymptomatic bacteriuria _____

5. abnormal blood glucose tolerance test _____

6. splenomegaly _____

7. urge incontinence _____

8. chronic bladder pain _____

9. hiccough _____

10. fever _____

11. ascites in the lower left quadrant of the abdomen _____

12. mass in epigastric area of abdomen _____

13. exanthem _____

14. nausea with vomiting _____

15. position dependent micturition _____

Provide two codes for each of the following diagnostic statements. Remember to list codes in the correct order, if it is specified.

16. elevated blood pressure and nervousness _____

17. pallor and flushing _____

18. gangrene due to diabetes _____

19. continuous urinary incontinence because of complete uterovaginal

    prolapse _____

20. precordial pain and hyperventilation _____

Provide the codes for the following case studies.

21. A patient's wife goes to the doctor with her husband. She is concerned about his excessive, deep sleep. Often, she is unable to wake him. She also mentions that her husband will stop breathing during these episodes and she lies awake waiting for him to start again. The patient is sent for sleep studies which show that he suffers from hypersomnia and sleep apnea.

    _____

22. A 63-year-old woman who experienced a stroke several weeks ago arrives to the office for a follow-up visit to determine the degree to which she has been affected by her stroke. After utilizing the National Institutes of Health Stroke Scale (NIHSS) to evaluate the impact of her stroke, the physician documents an NIHSS of 23. _____

23. A man comes in to the emergency department in excruciating pain. At this point he is not sure he can determine the origin of the pain, but it seems to be located in the back, high up on the right side. He is almost unable to walk and states the pain is worse than having a fractured bone. The ED physician suspects kidney stones, but until tests are done he documents renal colic. _____

24. A 30-year-old woman starts to notice that she can feel her heart beat in her chest. She is healthy, exercises, and cannot correlate these episodes with any activity or occurrence. She is seen by her physician who will set her up for laboratory studies and cardiac studies. Until he has those findings, he indicates a diagnosis of palpitations. _____

25. Patient has been exposed to HIV, is not symptomatic of the illness, but wants to be tested for the disease. His blood (serology) test comes back as nonspecific. _____

Injury, Poisoning and Certain Other Consequences of External Causes

Chapter 19: Codes S00–T88

Codes in the S-section of this chapter of ICD-10-CM classify injuries and wounds such as fractures, dislocations, sprains, strains, internal injuries, and traumatic injuries. Codes are organized by body region and type of injury, progressing from superficial through wounds to various types of fractures. Codes in the T-section of the chapter cover poisoning, burns, and many consequences of external causes. Often, external cause codes are also used to identify the cause of the injury or poisoning.

CODING TIPS

Laterality, Healing Stage, and Episode of Care for Injuries

Injury codes often employ sixth-position characters for laterality (right, left, or unspecified), and most codes in this chapter require an appropriate seventh-position character for the episode of care. Fracture documentation must supply the stage of healing for subsequent encounters, either normal healing or problems such as delayed healing, nonunion, or malunion.

The basic options are A for the initial encounter, D for a subsequent encounter, and S for sequela. In some cases, episode of care and fracture characteristics are combined in seventh-character choices, such as A for initial encounter for a closed fracture versus B for initial encounter for an open fracture.

Defaults for Fracture Coding

Classifications of fractures include whether they are open or closed and also displaced or not. In a closed fracture, the broken bone does not pierce the skin. An open fracture involves a break through the skin. If the fracture is not indicated as open or closed, code it as closed. A similar guideline applies to displaced versus not displaced fractures: lacking documentation, code to displaced.

Burns

Burns may require two codes: the first code for the burn's severity/body site, and for third-degree burns, a second code for its extent, known as total body surface area (TBSA). Burns are injuries that come from a heat source, while corrosions are burns due to chemicals.

1. Code current burns from categories T20–T25. These site/severity codes are grouped by sections of the body. Severity is one of three degrees: first-degree, in which the epidermis is damaged; second-degree, in which

both the epidermis and the dermis are damaged; and third-degree, in which all three layers of the skin are damaged. Assign a seventh digit to report the episode of care to further specify the site of the burn.

2. An additional code from categories T31 or T32 describes the TBSA involved based on the rule of nines (head and neck, 9%; each arm, 9%; each anterior leg, 9%; each posterior leg, 9%; anterior trunk, 18%; posterior trunk, 18%; genitalia, 1%). Study the illustration below. Note that TBSA codes are secondary when the burn site is specified, but primary when no site is specified.

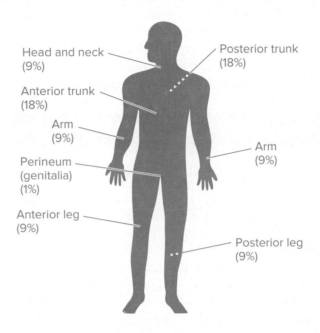

Provide the codes for the following diagnoses.

1. open fracture of nasal bones _____

2. closed fracture of sacrum and coccyx _____

3. unstable burst fracture of first lumbar vertebra _____

4. displaced fracture of left big toe _____

5. metacarpophalangeal joint sprain, thumb _____

6. strained sacroiliac ligament _____

7. concussion with 15-minute loss of consciousness _____

8. puncture wound of left front thorax wall, penetrating into thoracic cavity, subsequent visit _____

9. dislocation of the right side of the jaw _____

10. open wound of nasal septum _____

11. complicated wound of upper arm _____

12. black eye _____

13. injury to auditory nerve _____

Injury, Poisoning and Certain

continued

14. immediate shock after an injury _____

15. late effect of open animal bite on right knee _____

16. rupture of rotator cuff (traumatic) _____

17. closed posterior humeral dislocation _____

18. displaced Maisonneuve's fracture, left leg, follow-up visit, healing well ____

19. closed fracture of the acromial process, right shoulder _____

20. greenstick fracture, condylar process, left mandible _____

21. open fracture of base of skull _____

22. ruptured superior vena cava _____

23. posterior arch fracture of cervical vertebra, C1–C4 _____

24. fracture of distal phalanx of right thumb _____

25. pneumohemothorax _____

Provide the codes for the following case studies.

26. Patient went to the emergency department after a fall in his home. He tripped on a rug, and when he fell, the front of his neck hit the arm of his sofa. The area is very sore, and he is concerned that he may have further complications. He is examined, and the ED physician documents esophageal bruise. _____

27. A teenager practicing magic tricks is taken to the emergency room because he swallowed a nickel. The ED physician suggested he wait for nature to take its course. If that is not successful, he should see his own doctor at a later time. _____

28. After falling off his skateboard, the patient noticed a large bruise on one of his left toes. After waiting a few weeks after his initial appointment, the patient visited his physician to have the injury reexamined, as the pain persisted. The physician diagnosed a Salter-Harris type I physeal fracture of the phalanx of his left toe with delayed healing on this visit. _____

29. Patient presents with a portion of his left ear torn away after a motorcycle accident. The physician diagnosed left ear avulsion. _____

30. A 10-year-old girl comes to the ED. Her wrist is at an unusual angle, and she is in great pain. She was learning to skate for the first time and fell, using her hand to block her fall. X-rays are taken and the findings are that she has a fractured wrist. _____

Provide an injury code and an external cause code for each of the following diagnostic statements.

31. 7 ribs fractured due to fall from forklift truck _____

32. lacerations to hand from broken glass _____

33. forearm crushed under packing crate _____

34. bruise on buttock from fall during a horseback ride _____

35. snowblower accident caused multiple open wounds of lower limb

_____

Provide one or two codes for the following burns, as appropriate.

36. third-degree burns of face, head, and neck (*Hint:* Provide a code for the burn degree and location, and a code for the 9% TBSA third-degree burn.) _____

_____

37. first-degree burn of thigh and lower leg _____

38. second-degree chemical burn of palms _____

39. full-thickness skin loss of front and back of trunk _____

40. third-degree burns of both legs and upper and lower back _____

CODING TIP

Poisoning, Adverse Effects, and Underdosing

Poisoning refers to the medical result of the incorrect use of a substance. For poisonings, select the code based on intent (accidental, intentional self-harm, assault, and undetermined). Also code manifestations that are documented.

Poisoning is different from accidental harm caused by a reaction to the correct dosage of a drug, called adverse effects. For these situations, assign the appropriate code for the adverse effect and also use additional codes to report all manifestations, such as renal failure.

Underdosing, defined as taking less of a medication than prescribed, is coded from categories T36–T50.

The Table of Drugs and Chemicals following the Alphabetic Index lists these agents alphabetically, and Column 1 contains the code for the poisoning. Use the table first to point to a code that you verify in the Tabular List under categories T36–T65.

Identify the base codes for the following substances in the Table of Drugs and Chemicals.

41. carbitol _____

42. calomel _____

Injury, Poisoning and Certain
continued

43. iron compounds _____

44. Hexone _____

45. hornet sting _____

Provide the codes for the following diagnoses.

46. paralysis, black widow spider _____

47. ampicillin taken in error _____

48. overdose of levodopa _____

49. toxic effect of petroleum products _____

50. restenosis of peripheral vascular stent _____

51. intentional ingestion of rubbing alcohol _____

52. toxic effect, fumes of lead salts _____

53. patient unexpectedly gains awareness while under general anesthesia

    during a procedure _____

54. accidental hypothermia _____

55. heat prostration _____

56. toxic effect of lye _____

57. poisoning by topical dental drugs _____

58. poisoning from local anesthetic _____

59. late effect from displacement of implanted electronic neurostimulator,

    generator _____

60. methadone underdose _____

61. overdose of ovarian hormones _____

62. poisoning by coronary vasodilator _____

63. follow-up appointment due to the leakage of an indwelling urethral

    catheter _____

64. radiation sickness _____

65. anaphylactic shock after eating peanuts _____

Coding Quiz: ICD-10-CM

NAME _____

_____ **1.** Select the correct code for a personal history of cervical cancer.

    ① Z80.41
    ② C53.9
    ③ Z85.41
    ④ Z85.40

_____ **2.** Which is the correct code for a liveborn infant delivered by cesarean section in the hospital?

    ① Z37.0
    ② Z38.01
    ③ Z37.1
    ④ O34.219

_____ **3.** Select the correct code(s) for an ER visit for a patient who suffered a closed fracture of the head of the left radius in a fall from the moped he was driving on a highway.

    ① S52.122A
    ② S52.122B, V28.4XXA, Y92.411
    ③ S52.122A, V28.4XXA, Y92.411
    ④ S52.90XC, V41.5XXA, Y92.411

_____ **4.** Light-headedness after taking a diazoxide prescription:

    ① R42
    ② T46.5X2
    ③ H81.90
    ④ R42, T46.5X5A

_____ **5.** Select the correct code(s) for a plantar wart.

    ① B07.8
    ② B07.0
    ③ B97.7
    ④ B07.0, B97.7

_____ **6.** Acute bulbar type I infantile paralysis:

    ① A80.30
    ② A80.0
    ③ A80.39
    ④ A80.9

_____ **7.** Which code classifies intraductal cancer of the left female breast, upper-inner quadrant?

    ① D04.5
    ② C79.81
    ③ D48.62
    ④ D05.12

____ **8.** Screening test to rule out malignant neoplasm of the lung:

    ① Z12.2
    ② Z11.1
    ③ Z12.2, C34.90
    ④ C34.90, Z12.2

____ **9.** Select the correct code for a follow-up encounter due to delayed healing from a type II occipital condyle fracture.

    ① S02.111K
    ② S02.111G
    ③ S02.110G
    ④ S02.111A

____ **10.** A patient has been diagnosed with Burkitt's tumor in the groin and the neck. Select the correct code(s).

    ① C83.70
    ② C83.75, C83.71
    ③ C83.71, C83.75
    ④ C83.78

____ **11.** Select the correct code(s) for glaucoma and brittle type 2 diabetes.

    ① E11.9
    ② E11.39
    ③ E11.39, H40.839
    ④ E11.39, H40.9

____ **12.** Which of the following codes is correct for a diagnosis of abnormal coagulation profile?

    ① R79.1
    ② D68.9
    ③ R79.0
    ④ P53

____ **13.** Select the correct code for a neoplasm of unspecified behavior of the left kidney.

    ① D49.511
    ② D49.512
    ③ D41.012
    ④ D49.519

____ **14.** Which of the following correctly codes Alzheimer's disease with dementia and wandering off?

    ① F03
    ② G30.9, F02.81, Z91.83
    ③ G30.8
    ④ F02.81, G30.9, Z91.83

____ **15.** Select the correct code for a severe manic episode with psychotic features in manic-depressive disorder.

    ① F31.2
    ② F30.2
    ③ F30.9
    ④ F31.9

_____ 16. Choose the codes that correctly describe meningitis due to Lyme disease.

    ① A69.20

    ② A27.81

    ③ A69.21

    ④ G03.9

_____ 17. Lesions of the lateral and medial popliteal nerves:

    ① G58.9

    ② G57.30, G57.40

    ③ M54.30

    ④ G54.3, G54.4

_____ 18. An elderly female patient has been diagnosed with glaucomatous subcapsular flecks and open-angle glaucoma. Select the correct code(s).

    ① H40.10X0, H26.239

    ② H40.1194

    ③ H40.10X0

    ④ H26.239, H40.10X0

_____ 19. A 43-year-old male patient receives a diagnosis of essential hypertension and chronic endocarditis. Choose the correct code(s).

    ① I10

    ② I38

    ③ I11, I38

    ④ I10, I38

_____ 20. A 64-year-old female patient with a history of tobacco use is admitted to the hospital for an acute inferoposterior transmural infarction (right coronary artery). Select the correct code(s).

    ① I21.11

    ② I21,09

    ③ I21.11, Z87.891

    ④ Z87.891

_____ 21. Select the correct code(s) for a diagnosis of psychomotor deficit following an aneurysm the patient suffered several years ago.

    ① I69.819

    ② I69.813

    ③ I69.815

    ④ I72.9, I69.813

_____ 22. The patient's diagnosis is vesicoureteral reflux with nephropathy (without hydroureter) and chronic obstructive pyelonephritis due to _E. coli_ infection. Select the correct codes.

    ① N13.70, N11.0, B96.20

    ② N11.1, B96.20

    ③ N11.0, N13.70

    ④ N13.729, N11.1, B96.20

_____ **23.** Purulent pleurisy with bronchocutaneous fistula due to a bacterial infection:

① J86.9, B96.89
② J86.0, B96.89
③ J86.0
④ J86.9

_____ **24.** The patient arrives walking gingerly and the physician diagnosis a Tailor's bunion on his left foot. Select the correct code(s).

① M79.672, M21.622
② M21.612
③ M21.629
④ M21.622

_____ **25.** The patient is diagnosed with a recurrent gangrenous ventral hernia. Select the correct code(s).

① K43.1
② K43.9, I96
③ I96, K43.9
④ K43.1, I96

_____ **26.** Diverticulosis and diverticulitis of the small intestine with bleeding:

① K57.12
② K57.13
③ K57.12, K92.2
④ K57.11, K57.13

_____ **27.** A 58-year-old male patient has congenital stenosis of the vesicourethral orifice and urinary incontinence. Select the correct code(s).

① N32.0, N39.3
② Q64.31, R32
③ N32.0
④ R32

_____ **28.** A female infant 25 days old is light in weight for her age, weighed 1200 grams at birth, and has dry peeling skin. Select the correct code(s).

① P05.14
② P07.14
③ P05.04
④ P05.04, P04.5

_____ **29.** A pregnant patient in the twentieth week of gestation experiences bleeding that is resolved before delivery.

① O21.0
② O20.9
③ P15.9
④ O20.8

_____ **30.** Select the correct code(s) for erectile dysfunction after radiation therapy with left testicular pain.

① N52.39, N50.812
② N52.39, N50.82

③ N52.35, N50.812

④ N52.35, N50.82

_____ 31. A patient's diagnosis is periostitis and acute hematogenous osteomyelitis of the right femur caused by methicillin susceptible *S. aureus,* Group A. Choose the correct code(s).

① B95.0

② M86.051, B95.0

③ M86.051, B95.61

④ M86.051

_____ 32. An infant is diagnosed with spina bifida and hydrocephalus; its spinal column at C1 and C2 did not close during fetal development. Which code is correct?

① Q07.03

② Q05.0

③ Q05.5

④ Q05.2

_____ 33. Eighteen hours following the delivery of her baby, a female patient who has been discharged suffers atonic hemorrhage. Choose the correct code.

① O72.2

② O72.3

③ O72.1

④ P00.3

_____ 34. A 24-year-old female patient has a positive result from an HIV test; she is asymptomatic at the present. Which code is correct?

① B20

② Z11.59

③ Z21

④ Z11.51

_____ 35. A patient presents to the emergency room in some distress, complaining of precordial chest pain in the vicinity of the heart. The correct code is:

① R07.1

② R07.2

③ R07.89

④ R07.9

_____ 36. After an accident in which a car tire blows up, a patient suffers injuries to the saphenous vein and popliteal artery and vein. Select the correct codes.

① S85.309A, S85.009A, S85.509A, W37.8XXA

② W37.8XXA, S85.009A, S85.509A, S85.309A

③ S85.319A, S85.019A, S85.519A, W37.8XXA

④ S85.309A, S85.009A, S85.509A, W37.800A

_____ 37. A patient experiences a superficial sunburn on the eyelids. Select the correct code(s).

① T20.09XA W89.8XXA

② L55.9

③ T26.00XA, W89.8XXA

④ L55.0, X32.XXXA

_____ **38.** A patient has gastric hemorrhage following the unintentional ingestion of lye. Select the correct code(s).

① T54.3X1A, K92.2

② T54.3X2A, K92.2

③ K92.2, T54.3X4D

④ K92.2

_____ **39.** After having acute poliomyelitis as a child, a patient experiences muscle weakness diagnosed as postpolio syndrome. Select the correct code(s).

① M62.81, G14

② G14, M62.81

③ M62.81, B91

④ B91

_____ **40.** From a fire in a school, a patient has first-degree burns of the back of the right hand and third-degree burns of the left foot. Which codes are correct?

① X00.8XXA, T23.301A, T25.322, T31.21A

② T23.301A, T31.21A

③ T25.322A, T23.161A, T31.0, X00.0XXA, Y92.219

④ T30.0

Part 2 CPT and HCPCS

C PT, a publication of the American Medical Association that stands for Current Procedural Terminology, contains the codes mandated by HIPAA for professional services and procedures. These CPT codes also make up Level I of the Health Care Common Procedure Coding System (HCPCS) of the Centers for Medicare and Medicaid Services. Level II of HCPCS has codes to identify products, supplies, and services not covered in CPT. HCPCS is the HIPAA-mandated code set for Medicare and Medicaid services, and its Level II codes are also used by private payers.

The CPT manual contains three types of codes. Category I codes, which make up most of the book, describe the procedures and services that are commonly used in medical practice and performed by physicians in the United States. Category II codes are used for performance-measurement tracking. Category III codes are assigned as temporary codes for emerging technology, services, and procedures.

HCPCS and CPT codes are updated annually, except for Category II and III codes, which are updated twice a year. The CPT and HCPCS code sets are released midyear and take effect on January 1 of each year. HIPAA requires the correct codes to be used as of their effective date for reporting to all payers, both government and private.

CPT's main text, which contains the Category I codes, has these six sections of codes:

- Evaluation and Management   Codes 99201–99499
- Anesthesia   Codes 00100–01999
- Surgery   Codes 10021–69990
- Radiology   Codes 70010–79999
- Pathology and Laboratory   Codes 80047–89398
- Medicine   Codes 90281–99607

CPT codes have five digits (with no decimals) followed by a descriptor, which is a brief explanation of the procedure. Although CPT codes are grouped into sections, such as surgery, codes from any section can be used by all types of physicians. For example, a cardiologist would use codes from the Evaluation and Management Section when assessing a patient's suitability for a vascular procedure.

Locating Correct Codes

Medical coders follow a series of steps to choose correct procedure codes.

Step 1.
Determine the Procedures and Services Performed during the Encounter

The procedures and services performed during the patient's encounter with the provider are documented in the patient's medical record. The main procedure(s) provide(s) the descriptor to be coded first. Additional services or procedures are then coded.

Step 2.
Locate the Descriptor in the Index and Verify the Code Selection in the Main Text

Index

The index is used to find the descriptive term for the main procedure. The main terms in the index are printed in boldface type. The procedure may be listed more than once under these types of main terms:

- The name of the procedure or service
- The name of the organ or other anatomical site
- The name of the condition
- A synonym or an eponym for the term
- The abbreviation for the term

The index entry provides a pointer to the correct code range in the main text. Using the CPT index makes the process of selecting procedural codes more efficient. If the term is not located under a particular procedure or service, look next under alternate terms, such as *excision* instead of *removal*. Check also under the anatomical site or condition.

Main Text

The main text listing is reviewed to verify the selection of the correct code. Each of its six sections lists codes and descriptions under subsection headings. These headings group procedures or services, body systems, anatomical sites, or tests and examinations. Following these headings are additional subgroups of procedures, systems, or sites. The section, subsection, and code number ranges contained on a particular page are shown at the top of each page, making it easier to locate a code.

Note that each section begins with guidelines for the use of its codes. The guidelines cover definitions and items unique to the section, as well as special notes about its structure or the rules for its use. The guidelines must be carefully studied and followed for correct coding.

CPT uses a semicolon when a common part of a main entry applies to indented entries that follow. The descriptor that appears before the semicolon is the first part of a complete procedural description. Each descriptor that follows the

Section	Definition of Codes	Structure	Key Guidelines
Evaluation and Management	Physicians' services that are performed to determine the best course for patient care	Organized by place, type, and level of service	• New or established patients; other definitions • Unlisted services, special reports • Selecting an E/M service level
Anesthesia	Anesthesia services done by or supervised by a physician; includes general, regional, and supplementation local anesthesia	Organized by body site	• Time-based • Services covered (bundled) in codes • Unlisted services, special reports • Qualifying circumstances codes
Surgery	Surgical procedures performed by physicians	Organized by body system and then body site, followed by procedural groups	• Surgical package definition • Follow-up care definition • Add-on codes • Separate procedures • Subsection notes • Unlisted services, special reports
Radiology	Radiology services done by or supervised by a physician	Organized by type of procedure followed by body site	• Unlisted services, special reports • Supervision and interpretation (professional vs. technical components)
Pathology and Laboratory	Pathology and laboratory services done by physicians or by physician-supervised technicians	Organized by type of procedure	• Complete procedure • Panels • Unlisted services, special reports
Medicine	Evaluation, therapeutic, and diagnostic procedures done or supervised by a physician	Organized by type of service or procedure	• Subsection notes • Multiple procedures reported separately • Add-on codes • Separate procedures • Unlisted services, special reports

semicolon adds a unique word or words to complete the description. Note that the first letter of the common descriptor is capitalized, but the unique descriptors after the semicolon are not. Usually, the first unique entry appears in the same descriptor as the common part, and the other unique entries are indented below the first.

Resequenced Codes

As new procedures are widely adopted, CPT has encountered situations where there are not enough numbers left in a particular numerical sequence of codes for all the new items. Also, at times codes need to be regrouped into related procedures for clarity.

To handle this need, the AMA decided to resequence codes rather than renumbering and moving them. *Resequencing* means to display the codes in CPT out of numerical order so that they can be grouped according to the relationships among the code descriptions. It permits out-of-sequence code numbers to be inserted under the previous key procedural terms without having to renumber and move the entire list of related codes.

Codes that are resequenced are listed two times in CPT. First, they are listed in their original numeric position with the note that the code is now out of numerical sequence and refers the user to the code range containing the resequenced code and description.

Step 3.
Determine the Need for Modifiers

A CPT modifier is a two-digit number that may be appended to most five-digit procedure codes. Modifiers are used to communicate special circumstances involved with a procedure that are not adequately covered by the code descriptor. A modifier indicates to payers that the procedure was altered in some way that may affect the level of that code's reimbursement.

Applying Coding Guidelines

The CPT section of the *Medical Coding Workbook for Physician Practices and Facilities* is designed to build your skill in applying CPT coding guidelines. While following the organization of CPT, each section or subsection begins with a *Coding Tip* that explains important procedural coding rules, processes, or information. Some of these tips apply just to the particular CPT section which you are studying, and others apply globally when coding procedures and services. After completion of all the exercises in this part, you will know how to apply guidelines concerning:

- Modifier selection
- Bilateral and unilateral codes
- New and established patients
- Level of evaluation and management service—history, examination, and medical decision making
- Consultation versus referral
- Problems treated during preventive medicine services
- Anesthesia modifiers and qualifying circumstances codes
- Codes for add-on procedures
- Package codes and global periods
- Radiological supervision and interpretation
- Surgical procedures' inclusion of diagnostic procedures
- Separate procedures
- Procedures performed using various techniques or approaches
- Biopsies
- The obstetric package
- Procedures exempt from the 51 modifier
- Operating microscope
- Unlisted procedures and special reports
- Panels
- Injections
- Cardiac catheterization
- Category II code updates
- Category III code updates
- Locating correct HCPCS codes

Modifiers

A CPT modifier indicates that a procedure was different from the standard description, but not in a way that changed the definition or required a different code. Modifiers are used mainly when:

- A service or procedure was performed more than once or by more than one physician.
- Multiple procedures are reported on the same date of service.
- A service or procedure has been increased or reduced.
- Only part of a procedure was done. For example, some procedures have two parts—a technical component performed by a technician, and a professional component that the physician performed, usually the interpretation and reporting of the results. A modifier is used to show that just one of the parts was done.
- Unusual difficulties occurred during the procedure.

The modifiers are listed in Appendix A of CPT and in Appendix B of this workbook. However, not all CPT modifiers are available for use with every section's codes. Some modifiers apply only to certain sections. Two or more modifiers may be used with one code to give the most accurate description possible.

CODING TIP

Bilateral and Unilateral Codes

Some procedures have a pair of codes, one for a unilateral service and another for a bilateral service. Others are bilateral, applying to both anatomical parts or sections. For example, in the audiology section, the tinnitus assessment code 92625 describes a test of both ears. In other cases, codes are unilateral and require a 50 modifier when performed on both parts or sections.

If a procedure with a bilateral code is performed on just one of the two parts, a modifier is also needed. Use the 52 modifier, reduced services, to show that half the work described by the code was done.

Provide the correct modifier for each of the following descriptions.

1. multiple modifiers _____

2. distinct procedural service _____

3. unrelated Evaluation and Management Services by same physician during

   a postoperative period _____

4. staged procedure _____

5. assistant surgeon _____

6. discontinued procedure _____

7. repeat procedure by same physician _____

8. unusual anesthesia _____

9. mandated services _____

10. surgical team _____

11. surgeon administers a regional Bier block _____

12. patient hemorrhaged heavily during surgery; procedure took twice as long

    as typically required to perform _____

13. surgeon repairs the flexor tendon of the foot and excises a ganglion on the

    fourth toe _____

14. during an operation, a thoracic surgeon provides surgical access to the

    spine while an orthopedist performs a spinal fusion

    _____

15. surgeon provides part of a procedure _____

16. patient is returned to the operating room three hours after surgery because

    of ruptured sutures _____

17. This patient had been in Vermont skiing where he fractured his tibia.
    The surgery to repair the tibia was performed in Vermont. The patient
    was so anxious to get back home that he left the day after surgery and
    returned to his own orthopedist who did all the follow-up care. Code for
    this follow-up care.

    _____

    _____

18. After mammography findings of a density in both breasts, a patient
    undergoes puncture aspiration of a cyst in each breast.

    _____

    _____

19. A radiologist who is not employed by the hospital provides the report-
    ing function for all x-rays taken at the hospital. What modifier is used to
    reflect her services?

    _____

    _____

20. During the performance of a left lung lobectomy, a surgeon disconti-
    nues the surgery as he realizes the patient is going into shock during the
    procedure.

    _____

    _____

Evaluation and Management

Codes 99201–99499

The codes in the Evaluation and Management Section (E/M codes) of CPT cover physicians' services that are performed to determine the best course for patient care. Most codes are organized by the place of service. A few, such as consultations, are grouped by type of service. The subsections are as follows:

Office or Other Outpatient Services

Hospital Observation Services

Hospital Inpatient Services

Consultations

Emergency Department Services

Critical Care Services

Nursing Facility Services

Domiciliary, Rest Home (e.g., Boarding Home), or Custodial Care Services

Domiciliary, Rest Home (e.g., Assisted Living Facility), or Home Care Plan Oversight Services

Home Services

Prolonged Services

Case Management Services

Care Plan Oversight Services

Preventive Medicine Services

Non-Face-to-Face Services

Special Evaluation and Management Services

Newborn Care Services

Delivery/Birthing Room Attendance and Resuscitation Services

Inpatient Neonatal Intensive Care Services and Pediatric and Neonatal Critical Care Services

Care Management Services

Transitional Care Management Services

Advance Care Planning

Other Evaluation and Management Services

Many subsections list different code ranges for new and for established patients. A new patient has not received any professional services from the physician (or from another physician of the same specialty in the same group practice) within the past three years. An established patient has received professional services under those conditions.

In some medical practices, physicians assign E/M codes; in others, medical coders perform this task. In either case, code assignment should always be audited using a careful comparison between the codes that are reported and the procedures that are documented in the patient's medical record.

To select the correct E/M code, use the following eight steps.

Step 1.
Determine the Category and Subcategory of Service Based on the Location of Service and the Patient's Status

Step 2.
Determine the Extent of the History That Is Documented

The extent of the history that the physician obtains is one of four levels:

- Problem-Focused
- Expanded Problem-Focused
- Detailed
- Comprehensive

These components of history may be documented in the patient medical record:

- History of Present Illness (HPI)
- Review of Systems (ROS)
- Past Medical History (PMH)
- Family History (FH)
- Social History (SH)

The extent of history is determined according to the following table:

Extent of History	History of Present Illness	Review of Systems	Past/Family/ Social History
PROBLEM-FOCUSED	Brief	None	None
EXPANDED PROBLEM-FOCUSED	Brief	Problem-Pertinent	None
DETAILED	Extended	Extended	Problem-Pertinent
COMPREHENSIVE	Extended	Complete	Complete

Step 3.
Determine the Extent of the Examination That Is Documented

The physician may examine a particular body area or organ system, or conduct a multisystem examination. The examination is categorized as one of four levels:

- Problem-Focused—a limited examination of the affected body area or organ system
- Expanded Problem-Focused—a limited examination of the affected body area or organ system and other symptomatic or related organ system(s)
- Detailed—an extended examination of the affected body area(s) and other symptomatic or related organ system(s)
- Comprehensive—a general multisystem examination or a complete examination of a single organ system

Note that there are guidelines about the categories of examinations that are not printed in CPT. Called the **Documentation Guidelines for Evaluation and**

Management Services, they have important details used by physicians and medical coders to categorize the extent of examinations. Two sets of guidelines are currently approved for use, the 1995 and the 1997 versions. The 1997 set of guidelines, which is most commonly used, lists items that can be documented to satisfy the general multisystem examination requirements as well as items for each major medical specialty. The set of guidelines chosen by the medical practice should be specified and available to medical coders, along with other references.

Step 4.

Determine the Complexity of Medical Decision Making (MDM) That Is Documented

The complexity of medical decisions involves how many possible diagnoses or treatment options were considered; how much data (such as test results or previous records) were considered to analyze the patient's problem; and how much risk there is for significant complications, advanced illness, or death. The decisions that the physician makes are categorized as one of four types:

- Straightforward
- Low Complexity
- Moderate Complexity
- High Complexity

Complexity of Medical Decision Making	Diagnosis Options	Data Reviewed	Risks
STRAIGHTFORWARD	Minimal	Minimal or none	Minimal
LOW COMPLEXITY	Limited	Limited	Low
MODERATE COMPLEXITY	Multiple	Moderate	Moderate
HIGH COMPLEXITY	Extensive	Extensive	High

Step 5.

Analyze the Requirements to Report the Service Level

The descriptor for each E/M code explains the standards for its use. For office visits and most other services to new patients, and for initial care visits, all three of the key component requirements—history, exam, and MDM—generally must be met. For most services for established patients, and for subsequent care visits, two out of three of the key component requirements generally must be met.

Step 6.

Review the Nature of the Presenting Problem and the Time Spent with the Patient

Many descriptors mention two additional components: (1) how severe the patient's condition is—referred to as the "nature of the presenting problem" and (2) how much time the physician typically spends directly treating the patient. These factors, while not the key components, are helpful in selecting the correct service level.

Step 7.
Verify That the Documentation Is Complete

Meeting the requirements means that the documentation must contain the record of the physician's work. When an E/M code is assigned, the patient's medical record must contain the clinical details to support it. The history, examination, and medical decision making must be sufficiently documented so that the medical necessity and appropriateness of the service can be understood.

Step 8.
Assign the Code

The code that has been selected is assigned. The need for any modifiers, based on the documentation of special circumstances, is also reviewed.

CODING TIPS

Reimbursement for Consultations Depends on the Payer

A consultation occurs when a second physician provides services requested by the patient's primary physician and then returns the patient to that primary physician, with a written report of findings, to continue care. Referrals, on the other hand, involve the assumption of care by the physician to whom the patient is referred.

Because of suspected misuse of consultation codes, which reimburse at a higher rate than regular visits, CMS and many commercial payers have decided not to pay them. Coders coding for Medicare-paid (Original Medicare Plan) visits should use new/established patient codes for office/outpatient consultations and initial/subsequent hospital care codes for inpatient consultations.

Problems Treated during Preventive Medicine Service

An illness or clinical sign of a condition may be found during a routine physical examination that requires the physician to conduct an additional evaluation of the problem. In this case, the preventive medicine service code is reported first, followed by the appropriate E/M code for the new problem, adding the 25 modifier, Significant, Separate E/M Service.

Evaluation and Management
continued

Provide the procedure codes from the Evaluation and Management Section for the following procedures.

1. initial office visit, 25-year-old male, with boil on back; physician took a brief history, performed a limited examination of the back; there was little risk of complications and minimal treatment options

   _____

2. office visit, established patient is a 67-year-old female, with controlled diabetes mellitus, complaining of lack of sensation in her feet; expanded problem-focused history and examination

   _____

3. first hospital visit, admitting physician, comprehensive history, examination, and moderate decision making _____

4. initial office consultation, non-Medicare; detailed history and examination, low complexity medical decision making _____

5. annual comprehensive physical examination for 11-year-old new patient

   _____

6. medical disability examination by physician employed by state

   _____

7. hospital visit to previously admitted patient; problem-focused history and examination, 10 minutes spent at bedside _____

8. emergency department service for patient following a car accident; comprehensive history and examination, highly complex decision making

   _____

9. discharge of patient from nursing home, 45-minute encounter

   _____

10. home visit for established patient, straightforward case, problem-focused examination _____

11. While hospitalized for surgery, a non-Medicare patient takes a minor fall and hurts his elbow. An orthopedist is called in to consult to be sure injury is minimal. He determines it is a minor problem, and his visit is brief. _____

12. A patient is badly injured in a car accident and is put in an ambulance to get to the emergency department. On the way, his blood pressure drops and he has difficulty breathing. The EMT calls the ED physician who directs the care of the patient until they reach the hospital.

_____

13. A patient is admitted to the hospital in respiratory failure and kidney failure. He is sent to the intensive care unit where the ICU physician works on him for 1 hour to restore his breathing function and to dialyze him until he is stable.

_____

14. A child who is 25 days old was admitted 2 days ago to the neonatal intensive care unit due to cardiac and respiratory insufficiency. Today his physician is again monitoring his cardiac and respiratory support and reevaluating his status. The child has been under constant supervision by the health care team that is supervised by his physician.

_____

15. An 85-year-old woman fell and broke her hip. The hip has been repaired, but she now needs long-term nursing care. She was admitted to a nursing facility 3 days ago and is being seen today in follow-up. She is regaining movement and has an excellent prognosis.

_____

In addition to E/M codes, provide the modifiers and additional procedure codes if appropriate for the following procedures.

16. comprehensive annual examination for established 65-year-old patient

_____

17. Primary care physician sends a Medicare patient to a cardiologist for an evaluation of a complicated vascular problem; during the hour-long encounter, the specialist performs a comprehensive history and examination of this new patient, and follows up the visit with a written report to the PCP; MDM was moderate.

_____

18. Thoracic surgeon provides a second opinion on the appropriateness of a single bypass procedure as requested by a third-party payer; a detailed history and examination are obtained; MDM is of low complexity.

_____

19. During an annual physical examination, a 45-year-old established patient complains of general tiredness and severe shortness of breath during mild activity; physician performs a detailed cardiovascular assessment with additional detailed history; following complex MDM, the physician also schedules an immediate complete heart study.

_____

Anesthesia Section

Codes 00100–01999

The codes in this section of CPT are used to report anesthesia services performed by or supervised by a physician. These services include general and regional anesthesia, as well as supplementation of local anesthesia. A single code covers preoperative evaluation and planning, care during the procedure, and routine postoperative care. The subsections are organized by body site.

CODING TIP

Anesthesia Modifiers and Qualifying Circumstances Codes

Because the patient's health affects the difficulty of anesthesia services, a physical status modifier is added to the CPT anesthesia code. The patient's physical status—from P1 to P6—is selected from the listing in the Anesthesia Section Guidelines.

Standard modifiers 22, 23, 32, 51, 53, and 59 are also commonly used with anesthesia codes. Note that modifier 47, Anesthesia by Surgeon, is used by surgeons and appended to a surgical procedure code, not for services performed by anesthesiologists or anesthetists or supervised by surgeons.

A set of add-on codes, also listed in the guidelines, is used in addition to the procedural codes to report qualifying circumstances such as extreme age or emergency conditions.

Provide the CPT codes for the following anesthesia services. Do not code a physical status modifier for these services; focus on the anesthesia codes. *Hint:* All codes are in the Anesthesia Section.

1. cesarean delivery _____

2. arthroscopic procedures of the hip joint _____

3. transurethral resection of prostate _____

4. breast reconstruction _____

5. heart transplant _____

6. needle biopsy of thyroid _____

7. repair of cleft palate _____

8. cervical spine procedure _____

9. esophageal procedure _____

10. thoracoplasty _____

11. Patient presents with severe vaginal bleeding. Multiple malignant tumors are found, and the patient is scheduled for a radical hysterectomy. Code for the anesthesia. _____

12. A patient is experiencing lower abdominal pain, and her gynecologist suspects there is a problem in her uterus and/or fallopian tubes. He schedules a hysterosalpingography. Code for the injection procedure required to perform the hysterosalpingography. _____

13. Two months ago, this patient had abdominal surgery and now presents with pain in the left lower extremity. Examination reveals an embolus in the femoral artery, and surgery is performed to remove the embolus.

_____

14. After 6 months of shoulder pain, the patient sees her physician. He examines the patient and is concerned that there may be a tear in the shoulder joint ligament, but he cannot be sure without going in with a scope to examine the area. The diagnostic arthroscopy is performed. Code for the anesthesia. _____

15. A pregnant patient comes in to the hospital in labor. This is her first child, so the obstetrician is aware that her labor may be prolonged. She contacts anesthesia to provide a continuous epidural to cover this patient through her labor and vaginal delivery. _____

Provide the anesthesia codes and modifiers for the following services.

16. procedure on popliteal bursa, patient with mild systemic disease

_____

17. open procedure, sacroiliac joint, normal patient _____

18. major abdominal vessel procedure for patient with life-threatening

disease _____

19. plastic repair, cleft lip, 6-month-old _____

20. amniocentesis, healthy mother _____

21. spinal fluid shunting procedure on moribund patient _____

22. anesthesia is induced but blepharoplasty is canceled _____

23. amputation, ankle and foot, severely diabetic patient _____

24. emergency room appendectomy in the lower abdomen _____

25. diagnostic arthroscopic procedure of knee joint, mildly arthritic patient

_____

26. cardiac catheterization for patient with malignant hypertension

_____

27. removal of donated organs from brain-dead patient _____

28. pneumocentesis, eighty-year-old patient _____

Surgery Section

The Surgery Section of CPT has these subsections:

General

Integumentary System

Musculoskeletal System

Respiratory System

Cardiovascular System

Hemic and Lymphatic Systems

Mediastinum and Diaphragm

Digestive System

Urinary System

Male Genital System

Reproductive System Procedures

Intersex Surgery

Female Genital System

Maternity Care and Delivery

Endocrine System

Nervous System

Eye and Ocular Adnexa

Auditory System

Operating Microscope

The Surgery Section Guidelines contain both general information and a listing of the subsections that have unique special instructions. These notes should be carefully read before selecting codes from the procedures that follow them.

Many of the major system subsections are organized anatomically, covering body parts from head to toe. Within this organization, codes are listed in groups of related types of procedures. Typical groupings are:

- Incisions: procedures that involve cutting into, such as those with the ending *-otomy* or *-tomy* (for example, tracheotomy)
- Excisions: procedures that involve surgical removal, such as those with the ending *-ectomy* (for example, lumpectomy). Other terms are biopsy, resection, or removal; radical resection means total excision.
- Introduction or removal, amputation
- Repair/revision/reconstruction (*-orrhaphy, -oplasty*)
- Manipulation or reduction
- Fixation or fusion (*-opexy*)
- Endoscopic or laparoscopic procedures

Many surgical procedures can be performed in more than one way or via more than one approach. Open surgical procedures are performed by creating a surgical incision to access the site. For some of these, the alternative use of the endoscope permits a less invasive procedure. Endoscopic procedures frequently listed in the Surgery Section include laparoscopy, colonoscopy, bronchoscopy, esophagoscopy, and arthroscopy. These procedures are performed using endoscopic equipment. For example, a laparoscope is an endoscope designed to examine the contents of the peritoneum through a small incision. An arthroscope is an endoscope designed to view the interior of a joint. These are diagnostic endoscopic procedures; the instruments are also used for surgical procedures. Other open procedures may be endoscopically assisted. Coders study the terminology used to identify the technique that has been used.

Surgical destruction is usually a part of the surgical procedure and is not listed under a separate grouping.

Two codes for fine needle aspiration are listed before the first surgical subsection. These codes are general and apply to any body system.

General; Integumentary System

Codes 10021–19499

The two codes in the General subsection only cover fine needle aspiration with and without imaging guidance. The codes in the Integumentary subsection of CPT's Surgery Section cover procedures performed on the integumentary system, including the skin, subcutaneous and accessory structures, nails, and breast. Integumentary system services also include wound and burn repairs as well as skin grafts.

The guidelines for many groupings of procedures, such as paring, excision, or destruction, indicate which specific services are included. For example, shaving of lesions includes local anesthesia and chemical or electrocauterization of the wound. Such services cannot be reported in addition to the code for the procedure.

CODING TIP

Codes for Add-On Procedures

A plus sign (+) next to any code in CPT designates an add-on procedure that is commonly carried out in addition to a primary procedure. Add-on code descriptors usually use phrases such as "each additional" or "list separately in addition to the primary procedure." The add-on codes are also listed in CPT's Appendix D.

In reporting add-on codes, do not list them alone or modify them with a 51 modifier. There are many add-on codes in the Integumentary System subsection; exercises 21–25 provide practice.

Provide the integumentary system codes for the following procedures.

1. simple incision and removal of foreign body, subcutaneous tissue

   _____

2. complicated I&D, skin abscess _____

3. excision of benign lesion, 0.5-cm diameter, upper arm _____

4. excision of a 2.1-cm benign lesion from the foot _____

5. abrasion of a single lesion _____

6. cervicoplasty _____

7. rhytidectomy of glabellar frown lines _____

8. escharotomy _____

9. left breast reduction _____

10. breast reconstruction with free flap _____

11. Patient is having surgery for aberrant breast tissue on the right breast. Once started, the surgeon determines that a lumpectomy is required, and performs that procedure. _____

12. Patient presents with a 4.1-cm malignant lesion on the nose. Due to the location of the lesion and the depth of the lesion, the surgeon removes it by chemical destruction, instead of excision. _____

13. Patient is being treated for psoriasis. She now has severe psoriasis lesions that have not responded to oral medication. Today her physician will provide steroid injections into nine of those lesions.

    _____

14. Weeks after the excision of a malignant lesion, the patient was left with a defect too large to repair by simple closure. The surgeon elected to use a neurovascular pedicle flap to ensure that the defect would have adequate blood supply to heal correctly. _____

15. After observing that a spot on her upper leg had grown bigger, a patient saw her dermatologist. The dermatologist determined that she had a malignant 3.3-cm lesion which he biopsied and excised, followed by a simple closure. _____

Some of the following procedures require two codes and/or the use of a modifier.

16. excision of malignant lesions, 1.1 cm, upper arm; 0.1 cm, foot _____

17. split graft, 80 sq cm, lower leg, staged procedure on infant _____

18. surgical removal of excess skin and tissue, upper arm and hand _____

19. needle core biopsy of both breasts (not using imaging guidance) _____

20. preparation and insertion of custom breast implant 5 days after mastectomy, performed by the same physician _____

Hint: Each of the following procedures requires add-on codes.

21. abrasion, nine lesions _____

22. application of 200-sq-cm skin xenograft _____

23. laser destruction of four premalignant lesions _____

24. debridement of infected skin, 18 percent of body surface _____

25. complex repair of wound on trunk, 12 cm _____

Musculoskeletal System

Codes 20005–29999

The codes in this subsection of CPT's Surgery Section cover procedures performed on the musculoskeletal system. General procedures, such as wound treatments, excision services, and grafts, are listed first. Codes are then grouped by body site, beginning with the head and ending with the foot. Each body site has the same organization: incision, excision, introduction/removal, repair/revision/reconstruction, fracture/dislocation, manipulation, arthrodesis (fusion or fixation), amputation, and other procedures. Casts/strapping and endoscopy/arthroscopy are the final code groups in the subsection.

CODING TIP

Package Codes and Global Periods

A package is a group of related procedures and/or services included under a single code. As defined in CPT, a surgical package includes the operation itself, local anesthesia (injection of a metacarpal/digital block or topical anesthesia), and all routine follow-up services. For example, in the musculo-skeletal subsection, surgical package codes include the application and the removal of the first cast or traction device. Payers often add some preoperative services to their definition of a package.

Payers set a global period—a certain length of time for which the expected services are to be provided—for each package. During a global period, no packaged service is reimbursed in addition to the fee for the package code. After the global period ends, all services that are provided can be reported.

Some types of services are not considered to be routine follow-up and are reported during the global period. For example, complications or recurrences that arise after therapeutic surgical procedures are reported with appropriate modifiers (such as for repeat or related surgical procedures). Care for other illnesses, injuries, or conditions that are unrelated to the surgical procedure are also separately reported. In these cases, use a 24 or 79 modifier when an E/M service or a procedure performed during the global period is not related to the package and should be paid. Following a diagnostic procedure, services not related to the recovery from that procedure may be reported, even though the care may be related to the patient's underlying condition.

Provide the musculoskeletal system codes for the following procedures.

1. removal of body cast applied by another physician _____

2. primary repair of ruptured Achilles tendon _____

3. tendon sheath incision _____

4. closed treatment of fractured ulnar shaft _____

5. complete wrist arthrodesis _____

6. humeral osteotomy _____

7. closed treatment of sesamoid fracture _____

8. open treatment of talus fracture _____

9. I&D of foot bursa _____

10. removal of humeral and glenoid components of prosthesis _____

11. lateral elbow tenotomy, open with bone debridement _____

12. distal humeral sequestrectomy _____

13. reinsertion of spinal fixation device _____

14. insertion of a lumbar interlaminar distraction device with open decompression _____

15. radial and ulnar osteotomy _____

16. amputation of tip of right thumb with direct closure _____

17. percutaneous skeletal fixation of posterior pelvic ring dislocation

_____

18. trocar biopsy of rib _____

19. anterior capsulorrhaphy, transfer of coracoid process _____

20. surgical removal of prepatellar bursa _____

21. Nine months after a humeral fracture repair, a patient returns to his physician with pain in the fracture area. Unfortunately the patient had not returned prior to this time for fracture care follow-up and now has a nonunion of the humeral fracture. The surgeon does an iliac graft to repair the nonunion. _____

22. Patient with osteoarthritis has been treated medically for the erosion of cartilage in the hip for over 5 years. After extensive discussion with the surgeon, the patient agrees to have a total hip replacement procedure performed. The surgeon explains that the surgery requires replacement of the acetabulum and the proximal femur with a prosthesis.

_____

23. After a bicycle fall, a patient sought treatment for right hip pain. The orthopedist determined that the acetabulum (hip socket) was fractured, but that it could be treated with manipulation and skeletal traction, rather than doing an open procedure to correct the fracture.

_____

Musculoskeletal System *continued*

24. Concerned about the spread of the patient's osteomyelitis of the proximal humerus, the orthopedic surgeon performed a craterization of that bone in hopes of stopping any further spread of the infection.

   _____

25. A patient whose back was strapped due to severe muscle spasms fell off a ladder and was in extreme pain. It was late in the evening, and the patient went to the emergency department for evaluation and treatment. After removing the strapping that was already in place, the ED physician was able to determine that the patient had wrenched his back again, but there was no dislocation or fracture. The ED physician put replacement strapping on the patient and indicated that the patient should see his orthopedist in the morning for follow-up care.

   _____

Some of the following procedures require two codes and/or the use of a modifier.

26. bunionectomy with sesamoidectomy, left and right halluces _____

27. surgical exploration of chest wound with debridement and removal of

   foreign body _____

28. arthrodesis of sacroiliac joint, graft harvested _____

29. talectomy provided during global period of previous unrelated

   surgery _____

30. medial and lateral meniscectomy _____

31. closed treatment of ankle dislocation under anesthesia with percutaneous

   skeletal fixation _____

32. epiphyseal arrest of distal femur, proximal tibia, and proximal fibula

   _____

33. closed treatment of dislocated sternoclavicular joint and patella

   _____

34. synovial biopsy and diagnostic arthroscopy of hip _____

35. surgical arthroscopy, ankle, with removal of foreign body _____

Respiratory System

Codes 30000–32999

The codes in this surgical subsection of CPT cover procedures performed on the respiratory system. Codes are grouped by body site: the nose, accessory sinuses, larynx, trachea and bronchi, and lungs and pleura. Each body site is organized by the type of procedure as appropriate: incision, excision, repair, introduction, and endoscopic. Each site's procedural guidelines specify the included services.

CODING TIP

Coding Moderate (Conscious) Sedation

In previous editions of CPT, a symbol ⊙ (a bullet inside a circle) next to a code meant that moderate sedation was a part of the procedure. However, in CPT 2017, that feature has been replaced by a range of codes (99151–99157) for reporting when moderate sedation is performed. Under the new system, providers who perform moderate sedation with a procedure will be required to report the appropriate moderate sedation code in order to receive full payment. It is important to note that it will not be appropriate to report modifier 52 for reduced services with a procedure that is not performed with moderate sedation.

Provide the respiratory system codes for the following procedures. Include any necessary modifiers.

1. maxillectomy _____

2. maxillary sinus irrigation _____

3. total laryngectomy _____

4. unilateral medialization laryngoplasty _____

5. simple revision of tracheostoma _____

6. cervical tracheoplasty _____

7. parietal pleurectomy _____

8. extrapleural thoracoplasty _____

9. complex surgical removal of dermoid cyst from nose _____

10. lateral rhinotomy to remove object from nose _____

Some of the following procedures require two codes. *Hint:* For endoscopic procedures, read the notes before this code group carefully.

11. surgical thoracoscopy with excisions of pericardial and mediastinal

    cysts _____

12. surgical nasal/sinus endoscopy with maxillary antrostomy _____

13. planned tracheostomy on infant _____

14. hematoma drainage from nasal septum _____

15. laser destruction of two intranasal lesions, internal approach _____

16. sinusotomy, three paranasal sinuses _____

17. bilateral nasal evaluation using endoscope _____

18. direct diagnostic laryngoscopy and tracheoscopy with operating

    microscope _____

19. diagnostic nasal/sinus endoscopy with sphenoid sinusoscopy
    and inspection of interior nasal cavity, sphenoethmoid recess and
    turbinates _____

20. turbinate excision followed by intranasal antrotomy _____

21. A neonate, born several hours ago, develops respiratory distress and
    requires emergency endotracheal intubation. _____

22. A patient comes to the emergency department after a motor vehicle
    accident. The patient did not wear a seat belt and was injured when
    he hit the steering wheel. The doctors determined that his lung was
    deflated as a result of air accumulated in the thoracic cavity. They did
    a thoracentesis and inserted a tube to allow for the air to escape and the
    lung to reinflate. _____

23. After determining that the patient had developed lung cancer in both
    lobes of the right lung, the thoracic surgeon removed two lobes due to the
    extent of the cancerous tissue. _____

24. Years of chronic sinusitis had created a severe blockage of the ethmoid
    sinus cavity on the left side, discovered on CT exam. A sinus endoscopy
    was performed to remove tissue from the ethmoid sinus both anterior and
    posterior. _____

25. A patient with asthma since childhood now presents with increased
    difficulty breathing. A CT scan indicates an abnormality in the right
    middle lobe. To finalize this patient's diagnosis, a diagnostic bronchos-
    copy is performed. _____

Cardiovascular System

Codes 33010–37799

The codes in this surgical subsection of CPT cover procedures performed on the cardiovascular system. Codes are grouped in two large sections, the heart and pericardium followed by the arteries and veins. Cardiac procedures include placement of pacemakers/pacing cardioverter-defibrillators, surgery on the heart valves, and coronary artery bypass.

Many cardiac procedures include related procedures. For example, coronary artery bypasses include taking arteries or the saphenous vein graft from other body sites. Arterial and venous procedures, such as aneurysm repair, angioplasty, and catheter placement, include establishing blood inflow and outflow as well as arteriograms that the surgeon performs.

CODING TIP

Radiological Supervision and Interpretation

Often the physician supervises and interprets radiological imaging such as x-rays in the course of performing surgery. When the physician provides radiological supervision and interpretation (S&I), a professional component modifier (26) is attached to the radiology code that is reported with the surgery codes.

The appropriate radiology code or code range is mentioned with the associated surgery codes in CPT. If more than one code is mentioned, the coder turns to the Radiology Section and examines the listed codes to select the correct option. In some cases, separate codes are listed for the professional and the technical components of the service.

Note that the professional component modifier is not used if the physician owns the equipment, provides the supplies, and employs the technicians used for the radiological imaging. In that case, the physician is providing the complete service, and the modifier is not appropriate.

Provide the cardiovascular system codes for the following procedures. Include any necessary modifiers.

1. removal of permanent pacemaker pulse generator _____

2. mitral valve valvotomy, closed heart _____

3. coronary artery bypass using single venous graft _____

4. myocardial resection _____

5. repair of complete atrioventricular canal _____

6. saphenopopliteal vein anastomosis _____

7. carotid thromboendarterectomy _____

8. exploration of femoral artery _____

9. intravenous introduction of intracatheter _____

10. endovascular repair of visceral aorta and infrarenal abdominal aorta, two visceral artery endoprostheses _____

11. insertion of implantable intraarterial infusion pump _____

12. percutaneous transluminal mechanical thrombectomy, including dialysis circuit _____

13. insertion of transvenous electrode for dual chamber pacing cardioverter-defibrillator _____

14. aortic suture repair _____

15. repair of transposed great arteries by aortic pulmonary artery reconstruction _____

16. pulmonary artery embolectomy _____

17. sinus of Valsalva aneurysm repair with cardiopulmonary bypass

_____

18. ligation of secondary varicose veins, left and right legs _____

19. repair by division of patent ductus ateriosus in 10-year-old

_____

20. ring insertion and valvuloplasty, tricuspid valve _____

The following procedures may require two codes and/or the use of modifiers.

21. subcutaneous removal of pacing cardioverter-defibrillator pulse generator, electrodes removed by thoracotomy _____

22. subsequent pericardiocentesis with radiological S&I _____

23. relocation of skin pocket for pacemaker _____

24. aortic valve replacement using an allograft valve with cardiopulmonary bypass _____

25. coronary artery bypass with one arterial graft and three venous grafts

_____

Cardiovascular System *continued*

26. common carotid-ipsilateral internal carotid and axillary-axillary arterial
bypass with venous grafts _____

27. ultrasound as screening study for abdominal aortic aneurysm

_____

28. excision of infected abdominal graft, surgical care only _____

29. central venous catheter placed percutaneously in adult _____

30. routine venipuncture _____

Provide the codes for the following case studies.

31. Patient with two blocked coronary arteries is scheduled for coronary
artery bypass grafting; however, due to sudden tachycardia a single
chamber temporary pacemaker is inserted to stabilize the patient, and the
bypass surgery is rescheduled for the next day. Code for the temporary
pacemaker insertion.

_____

32. Patient presents for replacement of his pulmonary valve which was
determined to have a congenital anomaly. During the surgery the patient
develops ventricular tachycardia, and the operation is discontinued.

_____

33. Patient is examined due to shortness of breath, and angiography reveals
an embolus in the pulmonary artery. A surgeon is called in to perform an
embolectomy of the pulmonary artery. Code for the surgery.

_____

34. Patient is placed on heart/lung bypass, and the main pulmonary artery is
opened in order to remove the blockage and interior lining of the artery.
The artery is then sutured closed, and the pulmonary endarterectomy is
accomplished.

_____

35. Patient with a descending thoracic aneurysm is scheduled for surgery.
Despite the new endovascular procedures available to treat aortic
aneurysms, this patient's aneurysm is not amenable to the endovascular
treatment and will have to undergo an open repair of the descending aorta
using a Dacron graft.

_____

Hemic and Lymphatic Systems; Mediastinum and Diaphragm
Codes 38100–39599

Codes in these two surgical subsections of CPT cover procedures involving the spleen, bone marrow or stem cell transplantation, lymph nodes and lymphatic channels, the mediastinum, and the diaphragm.

CODING TIP

Surgical Procedures Include Diagnostic Procedures

As a general guideline, surgical procedures include diagnostic procedures. When a diagnostic procedure is the only service, it is reported. When the diagnostic procedure is followed by a surgical procedure, the diagnostic service is not reported. For example, a procedure such as a peritoneoscopy (laparoscopy examination of the peritoneum) to view and diagnose a condition is reported. However, if the diagnostic examination is followed by surgical laparoscopy (through the same scope and during the same surgical session), the diagnostic procedure cannot be separately reported. Note that a diagnostic laparoscopy as a separate procedure is located in the Digestive System subsection, code 49320.

Provide the codes for the following procedures. Include any necessary modifiers. In some cases, more than one code is required.

1. extensive drainage of lymphadenitis _____

2. injection procedure for identification of sentinel node _____

3. laceration repair, diaphragm _____

4. mediastinoscopy _____

5. needle biopsy of lymph node _____

6. axillary excision of cystic hygroma _____

7. pelvic lymphadenectomy _____

8. laparoscopic splenectomy _____

9. total splenectomy _____

10. autologous stem cell transplantation _____

11. injection for lymphangiography _____

12. repair of chronic traumatic diaphragmatic hernia _____

13. lymphangiotomy _____

14. insertion of cannula in thoracic duct _____

15. mediastinotomy with removal of object via cervical approach

    _____

16. injection procedure for splenoportography with radiological S&I

    _____

17. injection procedure for bilateral pelvic/abdominal lymphangiography with

    radiological S&I _____

18. An oncologist recommends that the patient undergo a procedure
    to determine what stage the cancer is in. The surgeon performs a limited
    lymphadenectomy of the aortic and splenic lymph nodes for staging.

    _____

    _____

19. Patient was in a car accident and suffered intraabdominal blunt trauma.
    Upon examination, the physician determined that the spleen had been
    lacerated or ruptured, and surgery was scheduled. A repair of the ruptured
    spleen was performed. The surgeon also did a partial splenectomy due to
    other damage found.

    _____

    _____

20. A 50-year-old patient who had a mastectomy 3 years ago now comes in
    with lumps under her arms and on her chest. Both a complete axillary
    lymphadenectomy and a regional thoracic lymphadenectomy must be
    performed.

    _____

    _____

Digestive System

Codes 40490–49999

The codes in this surgical subsection of CPT cover procedures performed on the digestive system. Codes are grouped by body site: lips, mouth, pharynx, esophagus, stomach, intestines, rectum, anus, liver, biliary tract, pancreas, and abdomen. Each body site is organized by the type of procedure, such as excision and repair.

Endoscopic procedures are listed under the esophagus, intestines, rectum, anus, and biliary tract. In keeping with coding principles, a surgical endoscopic procedure includes a diagnostic endoscopic procedure.

CODING TIP

Separate Procedures

Some surgical code descriptors in CPT are followed by the words *separate procedure* in parentheses. These procedures are usually integral parts of the major procedure performed during an operation and therefore are not reported.

In some situations, however, a separate procedure is not done with the major procedure. It is performed alone and coded in the normal way. When a separate procedure is done along with other procedures but for a separate purpose, it may be reported in addition to the major operation code. In this case, the 59 modifier is attached to the separate procedure code to show that it is not a part of another procedure and is distinct and independent.

Provide the codes for the following procedures. Include any necessary modifiers. In some cases, more than one code is required.

1. resection of 50 percent of lip _____

2. repair of sliding inguinal hernia _____

3. insertion of peritoneal-venous shunt _____

4. exploratory laparotomy _____

5. removal of esophageal sphincter augmentation device _____

6. cholecystectomy with cholangiography _____

7. rigid esophagoscopy with specimen collection _____

8. wedge biopsy of liver _____

9. excision of Meckel's diverticulum _____

10. gastroduodenostomy _____

11. frenotomy _____

12. palate resection, repeated procedure by same physician _____

13. secondary adenoidectomy, 10-year-old patient _____

14. near total esophagectomy w/pharyngogastrostomy (w/o thoracotomy)

_____

15. percutaneous placement of gastrostomy tube w/radiological S&I

_____

16. endoscopic directed placement of gastrostomy tube w/radiological S&I

_____

17. simple ileostomy revision done during same operative session as pharan-
    geal wound suture _____

18. partial colectomy with ileostomy and creation of mucofistula _____

19. excision of ruptured appendix _____

20. diagnostic and surgical flexible colonoscopy past the splenic flexure and
    tumor removal by bipolar cautery _____

21. The physician does an endoscopic diagnostic evaluation of the patient's
    esophagus and stomach. The scope does not go beyond the cardia of the
    stomach.

    _____

22. Due to a patient's encroaching tumor, the surgeon removes half of the
    patient's tongue (hemiglossectomy).

    _____

23. Patient comes in 1 year after repair of his right and left incarcerated
    femoral hernias with a recurrence of that condition. The surgeon schedules
    surgery to repair this recurrent problem. Code for the surgery.

    _____

24. The patient's esophageal cancer has made it almost impossible for
    him to eat normally, and he is becoming malnourished. His physician
    recommends laparoscopically creating an opening into the jejunum
    (2nd portion of the small intestine) to allow for placement of a feeding
    tube. A laparoscopic jejunostomy is performed.

    _____

25. As a result of spasms in the esophagus, the patient is unable to swallow.
    The physician will need a greater than 35-mm balloon dilator to alleviate
    this patient's difficulty. Radiologic supervision and interpretation are
    provided via fluoroscopy using the hospital's equipment.

    _____

Urinary System
Codes 50010–53899

The codes in this surgical subsection of CPT cover procedures performed on the urinary system. Codes for the kidneys, ureters, bladder, and urethra are listed by the type of procedure. Different codes for males and females are indicated in some bladder and urethra procedures.

Many procedures involving the urinary system involve the use of a laparoscope or an endoscope. They include renal and ureteral laparoscopy and endoscopic procedures, cystoscopy (to view or treat the bladder), urethroscopy (to view or treat the urethra), and cystourethroscopy (using both the cystoscope and the urethroscope to view or treat the urinary collecting system). Therapeutic (surgical) procedures include diagnostic procedures as well as other listed procedures.

CODING TIP

Procedures Performed Using Various Techniques or Approaches

In researching codes in CPT, it is useful to be aware that some procedures are performed using different techniques. For example, a sling operation for stress incontinence may be performed as a surgical repair or laparoscopically. Some procedures are done by more than one method. For example, injections can be subcutaneous/intramuscular, intraarterial, or intravenous, each having a code. Carefully examine the description of the procedure to determine which technique or approach has been used before researching the code.

Provide the codes for the following procedures. Include any necessary modifiers. In some cases, more than one code is required.

1. ureterotomy _____

2. ureteroplasty _____

3. ureteral endoscopy through established ureterostomy _____

4. first-stage urethroplasty _____

5. drainage, deep periurethral abscess _____

6. cystourethroscopy with double-J type stent _____

7. closure of cystostomy _____

8. EMG studies of urethral sphincter _____

9. trocar bladder aspiration _____

10. simple bladder irrigation _____

11. ureteroileal conduit and Bricker operation _____

12. laparoscopic nephrectomy _____

13. percutaneous needle renal biopsy with radiological S&I (fluoroscopy)

    _____

14. complicated Foley Y-pyeloplasty _____

15. renal endoscopy through nephrotomy _____

16. completion (second stage) of transurethral prostate resection *Hint:* Include
    a modifier. _____

17. cystourethroscopy with fulguration of 3.0-cm bladder tumor _____

18. unilateral ureteroneocystostomy and cystourethroplasty _____

19. transurethral resection, obstructive tissue, 18 months after a TURP

    _____

20. discontinued contact laser vaporization of prostate _____

21. A urologist pulverizes a patient's kidney stones in the right kidney via
    lithotripsy (using shock waves directed through a water cushion). Over the
    next several days/weeks, the fragments will pass harmlessly through the
    urinary system. _____

22. A patient has been diagnosed with kidney failure and will need to go on
    dialysis until a kidney transplant is possible. Due to various difficulties
    with the patient's existing kidneys, both must be removed prior to the
    transplant. Code for their removal. _____

23. A urologist needs to examine both ureters and the bladder. She inserts a
    scope into the ureters making an incision in the opening of the ureters to
    the bladder (meatotomy) and completes the examination.

    _____

24. A 70-year-old patient was seen for chronic urinary urgency. The
    urologist's examination revealed an enlarged prostate that was most
    likely the cause of the problem. Testing determined that the patient
    did not have prostate cancer, and drug therapy was prescribed initially.
    The patient's problem was not alleviated, and surgery was recom-
    mended. The urologist performed an electrosurgical resection of the
    prostate, using a transurethral approach and internal urethrotomy.

    _____

25. After having given birth to four children and having a hysterectomy
    performed in her fifties, the 65-year-old patient presents today because she has
    problems retaining her urine when walking, sneezing, or coughing. She is
    embarrassed and wants the problem corrected. Her urologist recommends
    a sling operation to give her bladder support, and he recommends doing it
    laparoscopically. The patient agrees. Code for the surgery that will be
    performed. _____

Male Genital System; Reproductive System Procedures; Intersex Surgery

Codes 54000–55980

The codes in the male genital system surgical subsection of CPT cover procedures performed on the male genital system. Codes for the penis, testis, epididymis, tunica vaginalis, scrotum, vas deferens, spermatic cord, seminal vesicles, and prostate are listed by type of procedure. The only code in the reproductive system procedures subsection covers the placement of needles or catheters into pelvic organs and/or genitalia. Intersex codes cover male-to-female and female-to-male operative procedures.

CODING TIP

Biopsies

Codes for biopsies are located in many of the surgical subsections. Biopsies are performed with a number of different techniques, such as needle core, punch, incisional, or fine needle aspiration. In general, biopsies of all types follow the coding principle that surgical procedures include diagnostic procedures. If a biopsy is the only service performed, it is reported. As a general rule, however, if more extensive surgery is performed in addition to the biopsy, then the biopsy procedure is not reported with the major surgical procedure. Biopsies are often separate procedures in CPT.

Provide the codes for the following procedures. Include any necessary modifiers. In some cases, more than one code is required.

1. testicular injury repair _____

2. bilateral simple orchiectomy _____

3. bilateral vasectomy _____

4. complicated vesiculotomy _____

5. laparoscopic orchiopexy _____

6. radical perineal prostatectomy _____

7. excision of Mullerian duct cyst _____

8. ligation of vas deferens _____

9. removal of foreign body, scrotum _____

10. I&D, abscess of epididymis _____

11. fixation of contralateral testis _____

12. incisional biopsy of testis followed by radical orchiectomy for tumor, inguinal approach _____

13. simple electrodesiccation of four lesions on penis _____

14. surgical excision of papilloma on penis, extensive procedure _____

15. spermatocele excision _____

16. spermatic vein ligation for varicocele, discontinued service _____

17. spermatic vein ligation for varicocele, laparoscopic surgery _____

18. clamp circumcision of newborn _____

19. corpora cavernosography with radiological S&I _____

20. deep penile I&D _____

21. Cecil repair, third stage _____

22. repair, hypospadias cripple _____

23. After undergoing a hypospadias repair 2 months ago, the patient injured his penis during a basketball game and was operated on in order to repair it.

_____

_____

24. Patient presents with symptoms of deformity of his penis and painful erection. The physician diagnosed Peyronie's disease and performed an injection and then excision of penile plaque.

_____

_____

25. Patient had suffered from frequent urination, pressure, and pain in the bladder. Upon examination, the physician found a prostate mass. Due to the size and specific location of the mass, an incisional biopsy of the prostate was performed to determine if the mass was benign or malignant.

_____

_____

Female Genital System; Maternity Care and Delivery

Codes 56405–59899

The codes in these surgical subsections of CPT cover procedures performed on the female genital system and for maternity care and delivery. In the female genital system, codes for body site and for in vitro fertilization are listed by the type of procedure.

The maternity care and delivery codes have a unique organization. They are grouped as follows: antepartum services; excision; introduction; repair; vaginal delivery, antepartum and postpartum care (normal uncomplicated cases); cesarean delivery; delivery after previous cesarean delivery; abortion; and other procedures.

CODING TIP

The Obstetric Package

The guidelines for maternity care/delivery describe the obstetric package of services normally provided for uncomplicated cases. The package consists of antepartum care, delivery, and postpartum care, as described. Before coding obstetrical services, study these notes carefully to avoid unbundling—improperly reporting work that is part of the package. Understanding the obstetric package also permits correct reporting of those services that are not part of the package and that can be coded separately.

Provide the codes for the following procedures. Include any necessary modifiers. In some cases, more than one code is required.

1. simple destruction of four lesions, vulva _____

2. complete radical vulvectomy _____

3. fitting and insertion of pessary _____

4. laser destruction of vaginal lesions (simple) _____

5. D&C, cervical stump _____

6. D&C, postpartum hemorrhage _____

7. uterine suspension _____

8. total abdominal hysterectomy _____

9. subtotal hysterectomy _____

10. insertion of IUD _____

11. routine obstetric care/vaginal delivery, previous cesarean delivery

_____

12. missed abortion surgically completed in first trimester _____

13. abortion induced by D&C _____

14. cesarean delivery, surgical care only _____

15. cesarean delivery, including postpartum care, and total hysterectomy following attempted vaginal delivery; patient had previous cesarean delivery _____

_____

16. Strassman type hysteroplasty and closure of vesicouterine fistula

_____

17. chromotubation of oviduct including materials _____

18. laparoscopic assisted vaginal hysterectomy (uterus less than 250 grams) _____

19. multifetal pregnancy reductions _____

20. episiotomy by assisting physician _____

21. Making a small abdominal incision, the physician drains a cyst from each ovary. _____

22. An elderly woman without any prior history of cancer is diagnosed with an extensive malignant vaginal cancer, requiring vaginectomy and complete removal of the vaginal wall.

_____

23. An obstetrician has been seeing this patient starting with her first visit to determine that she is pregnant. She recently performed the vaginal delivery, and the patient is now being seen in the office for her last postpartum visit. How will the obstetrician code for her services?

_____

24. Patient has a hysterotomy to remove a hydatidiform mole as well as tubal ligation during the same surgical session.

_____

25. A patient is pregnant with her fourth child and is having contractions that are rapidly coming closer together. She and her husband leave for the hospital, but the baby is born in the car before reaching the hospital. Once the baby is secured by emergency medical technicians, the patient is admitted and her physician delivers the placenta.

_____

Endocrine System; Nervous System

Codes 60000–64999

The brief endocrine system subsection of the CPT Surgery Section contains codes for procedures on the thyroid gland, parathyroid, thymus, adrenal glands, and carotid body. The nervous system subsection comprises codes for nerves located in the skull, meninges, and brain; spine and spinal cord; extracranial nerves, peripheral nerves, and autonomic nervous system. Like the cardiovascular system section, the nervous system codes are complex, based on the particular anatomy and procedures required. Advances in techniques such as deep brain stimulation and pain management often lead to new and revised procedural codes in this section.

CODING TIP

Procedures Exempt from the 51 Modifier

In addition to add-on procedures or services, there are other procedures in CPT with which a 51 modifier for multiple surgical procedures cannot be used. The 51 modifier identifies additional surgical procedures that are done during the major, or primary, surgery. The primary procedure is paid in full, and the additional procedures automatically receive reduced payment. Modifier 51 exempt codes are identified with the symbol ⊘.

Provide the codes for the following procedures. Include any necessary modifiers. In some cases, more than one code is required.

1. total thyroid lobectomy _____

2. twist drill hole for subdural puncture _____

3. resection of a vascular lesion at the base of the posterior cranial fossa

   _____

4. craniotomy for repair of dural/CSF leak _____

5. exploratory craniectomy _____

6. aspiration of thyroid cyst _____

7. laparoscopic adrenalectomy _____

8. bilateral chemodenervation of neck muscles, excluding the muscles of the larynx _____

9. total thyroidectomy, limited neck dissection, for excision of malignancy

_____

10. adrenalectomy _____

11. injection of diagnostic anesthetic into lumbar via interlaminar epidural _____

12. epidural percutaneous implantation of neurostimulator electrodes

_____

13. implantation of cranial nerve neurostimulator electrodes

_____

Provide the codes and decide whether to append the 51 modifier.

14. craniectomy, infratentorial, to excise a brain abscess, and twist drill hole to implant ventricular catheter _____

15. vertebral corpectomy with decompression of spinal cord, three segments _____

16. A 57-year-old patient who had suffered from muscular tremors due to Parkinson's disease was treated with an intracranial neurostimulator. She now needs to have the electrodes removed, and surgery is performed to remove them. _____

17. A young patient was born with hydrocephalus due to the accumulation of cerebrospinal fluid (CSF) in the ventricles of his brain. He is now scheduled for surgery to allow the neurosurgeon to create/implant a shunt that will drain the CSF into the peritoneum, thereby relieving the pressure on the brain. _____

18. After months of back pain, a patient is scheduled for an MRI scan of the spinal cord. The scan shows a lesion in the thoracic spine near T1 and T2. The physician performs a percutaneous needle biopsy of the spinal cord, using CT scan for the radiological supervision and interpretation of the needle placement. _____

19. The lamina of the lumbar spine at L3 and L4 are compressing the spinal cord, causing great pain. The surgeon explains that she will remove a portion of lamina at both segments to decompress the spinal cord, but there will be no removal of the vertebral facets, disks, or a foraminotomy. The surgeon had previously determined that the compression problem is not caused by spondylolisthesis. _____

20. The discovery of an intracranial abscess located above the tentorium and another below the tentorium leads to the performance of a craniectomy to drain each abscess. _____

Eye and Ocular Adnexa; Auditory System; Operating Microscope

Codes 65091–69990

Codes in these subsections of CPT's Surgery Section are used to report surgical procedures on the eye, its surrounding structures, and the ear. Ophthalmological diagnostic and treatment services are not coded from the Eye and Ocular Adnexa codes. Use the Ophthalmology codes in the Medicine Section instead.

CODING TIP

Operating Microscope

An operating microscope—code 69990—is used in the performance of delicate surgical procedures. In some cases, CPT permits reporting of the operating microscope; in other cases, its use is always part of the procedure, and it cannot be reported in addition to the operation. For example, a note at the beginning of the eye and ocular adnexa subsection states that the operating microscope should not be reported in addition to codes 65091 to 68850—that is, with all the codes in this subsection. Be sure to review all notes when selecting codes.

Provide the codes for the following procedures. Include any necessary modifiers. In some cases, more than one code is required.

1. removal of embedded foreign body, eyelid _____

2. biopsy, conjunctiva _____

3. ear piercing _____

4. removal, electromagnetic bone conduction hearing device, temporal bone

   _____

5. complete mastoidectomy _____

6. canthotomy _____

7. closure of eyelids by suture, temporary _____

8. scleral reinforcement without graft _____

9. extracapsular cataract removal with insertion of intraocular lens prosthesis, mechanical technique _____

10. excision of scleral lesion _____

11. chalazion excision during the global period of a strabismus surgery

_____

12. tympanic membrane repair with operating microscope _____

13. biopsy of both external ears _____

14. impacted cerumen removed from both ears _____

15. ocular implant removal with operating microscope _____

16. removal of dislocated intracapsular lens _____

17. discontinued myringoplasty _____

18. biopsy and excision of exostoses from external auditory canal _____

19. tympanic neurectomy of both ears via suction _____

20. canthus reconstruction, surgical care only _____

21. A 70-year-old patient with chronic glaucoma is still suffering from elevated intraocular pressure that has not responded to medical therapy. To treat the problem surgically, the surgeon will have to destroy portions of the ciliary body to bring down the intraocular pressure. The surgeon elects to do this with a freezing probe (cryotherapy) to destroy the ciliary process. _____

22. This patient has been nearsighted all his adult life. Neither glasses nor contact lenses have sufficiently alleviated the problem, and the patient elects to have surgery. After applying topical anesthetic, the surgeon makes radial incisions on the anterior surface of the cornea, thereby flattening the cornea and correcting the refractive state. _____

23. A patient suddenly suffers from loss of vision in the right eye and goes to see the ophthalmologist. The examination shows that the retina of the right eye has detached and fallen into the posterior chamber of the eye causing loss of blood supply to the retina. The problem can be corrected with a retinal detachment repair by photocoagulation. The first repair is done the next day, and two more repairs are scheduled to be done within a 2-month treatment period. Code for the retinal detachment repairs. _____

24. The lacrimal sac, which is part of the lacrimal system that produces tears, has an abscess that must be drained in order for the lacrimal system to function properly. The surgeon makes a small incision directly into the lacrimal sac, and the pressure caused by the abscess is relieved as the area drains. The incision is sutured closed. _____

25. A senile elderly patient in a nursing home placed an earring in her ear which is now lodged in the external auditory canal. The patient's tendency to flail her arms whenever she is examined requires that general anesthesia be used to extract the earring. Once the patient has been anesthetized, the physician is able to visualize the earring and extract it with forceps and suction. _____

Radiology Section

Codes 70010–79999

The codes in the Radiology Section of CPT are used to report radiological services performed by or supervised by a physician, such as interpreting x-ray, ultrasound, and other types of imaging tests, and interventional radiology (image-guided surgery), in which diseases are treated nonoperatively using small catheters or other devices guided by radiological imaging. Codes in the diagnostic radiology and diagnostic ultrasound subsections are grouped anatomically. Radiation oncology and nuclear medicine subsection codes are arranged by service type.

Almost all radiology procedures have two parts: (1) a technical component, covering the technologist, the equipment, and processing, and (2) a professional component that includes the reading of the radiological examination and the physician's written interpretation report.

CODING TIP

Unlisted Procedures and Special Reports

Because of advances in medical knowledge and techniques, a new procedure may not have a Category I or a Category III code. Such procedures are reported using "unlisted" codes in each section. The unlisted procedure codes, which always end in 99 (for example, 79999), are printed in the section guidelines and also appear at the ends of their code sections.

Advances are especially common in the area of radiology services with the introduction of newer, faster, and better imaging technology. CPT has codes for 16 unlisted code areas in radiology. When unlisted codes are reported, a special report must be attached that defines the nature of, extent of, and need for the procedure, and describes the time, effort, and equipment necessary to provide it.

Provide the radiology codes for the following procedures. Do not include the 26 modifier. In some cases, more than one code is required.

1. radiologic examination of the ribs, two views (unilateral) _____

2. orthodontic cephalogram _____

3. magnetic resonance imaging of the pelvis (with contrast) _____

4. thoracic spine computerized tomography w/o contrast material _____

5. x-ray examination of the abdomen, single anteroposterior view _____

6. antegrade urography, S&I _____

7. serialographic thoracic aortography, S&I _____

8. complete study, cardiac MRI for function _____

9. ultrasound, scrotum _____

10. unilateral adrenal angiography, S&I _____

11. CT bone density study and limited osseous survey _____

12. bilateral screening mammography _____

13. unlisted radiopharmaceutical therapeutic procedure _____

14. PET tumor imaging, whole body _____

15. SPECT myocardial imaging _____

16. diagnostic nuclear medicine procedure, gastrointestinal, unlisted

_____

17. ten determinations of thyroid uptake _____

18. high-dose-rate brachytherapy, remote afterloading, 11 channels _____

19. repeated Doppler echocardiography, fetal cardiovascular system _____

20. red cell survival study _____

21. To confirm the diagnosis of a rotator cuff tear, the physician first anesthetizes the shoulder area and then, with a needle, injects contrast into the shoulder joint in order to visualize the area while taking a series of x-rays and interpreting what is found. Code for the physician's radiological supervision and interpretation of the x-rays. _____

22. After examination and testing by her internist, a young woman is still left with constant pelvic pain that cannot be diagnosed. The internist sends her for a CT scan with contrast to diagnose the problem. _____

23. An older construction worker developed eye pain after his sandblaster malfunctioned. He thought it was just "something in my eye," but after 4 hours he was still in great pain and was seen by his ophthalmologist. The ophthalmologist examined the eye, but had difficulty determining what was in the eye due to an early cataract in the affected eye. The patient was sent for an ophthalmic ultrasound to find what foreign body was causing the problem. _____

24. One of the services provided by a radiation oncologist to patients who are receiving radiation therapy for cancer is clinical treatment planning. Code for the clinical treatment planning that encompasses a single treatment area in a single port with no blocking. _____

25. A radiation oncologist reviews the port films, dosimetry, dose delivery, and treatment parameters, and also does a medical evaluation for a patient who receives eight treatments over 2 weeks. Code for the radiation oncologist's services related to the eight treatments. _____

Pathology and Laboratory Section
Codes 80047–89398

The codes in the Pathology and Laboratory Section of CPT cover services provided by physicians or by technicians under the supervision of physicians. These codes represent the services associated with performing the test and with analyzing and reporting the test results.

The codes are organized by the type of test: organ or disease oriented panels, drug testing, therapeutic drug assays, evocative/suppression testing, pathology consults, urinalysis, chemistry, hematology and coagulation, immunology, transfusion medicine, microbiology, anatomic pathology, cytopathology and cytogenetic studies, surgical pathology, and other procedures.

Note that since multiple procedures are commonly done on the same date of service, the 51 modifier is not used with codes from this section.

CODING TIP

Panels

Individual tests that are customarily ordered together are grouped under laboratory panels. When a panel code is used, all the listed tests must have been performed. If not, the codes for the separate component tests that were done should be reported instead of a panel code. If a panel code is reported, no individual test within it may be additionally reported, but other tests outside it may be reported. Do not report panels with overlapping tests. In this case, report the panel with the greater number of performed tests, and report the other tests using individual test codes.

Provide the pathology and laboratory codes for the following procedures. Include any necessary modifiers. In some cases, more than one code is required. *Hint:* Check the required components of the organ/disease-oriented panels when coding multiple tests.

1. total serum cholesterol _____

2. blood creatinine _____

3. three-specimen GTT _____

4. FSH gonadotropin test _____

5. vitamin K test _____

6. Saccomanno technique _____

7. hepatitis C antigen, direct probe _____

8. commercial-kit urine culture _____

9. Rh blood typing _____

10. EA test for Epstein-Barr virus _____

11. urine specific gravity, automated, no microscopy _____

12. RPR, quantitative _____

13. gabapentin assay _____

14. *SEPT9* methylation analysis _____

15. cholesterol, HDL, triglycerides, LDL _____

16. rubella screen _____

17. cryopreservation of five cell lines _____

18. HGH antibody _____

19. comprehensive clinical pathology consultation with report _____

20. drug screening for alcohols _____

21. A patient who had experienced chest pain and took a stress test has an abnormal reading. The cardiologist suspects a blockage in the coronary arteries and does a cardiac catheterization. This test shows the arteries are clear, but the aortic valve has an anomaly and has to be replaced. One of the tests the hospital will need both before and after surgery is the test that shows how long it takes for the blood to clot (bleeding time). Code for this test. _____

22. After his most recent chemotherapy treatment, a patient was quite weakened. His oncologist ordered a complete CBC. _____

23. A patient with chronic edema despite years of treatment with diuretics is considered to have a pituitary gland problem that may be secreting excessive amounts of vasopressin, an antidiuretic hormone. Code for the ADH test. _____

24. A patient presents with a 2-year history of urinary incontinence and pain when urinating. An examination shows an enlarge prostate gland, and his urologist now requests a test to check for the level of PSA, total.

_____

25. A young woman with a family history of high cholesterol is now pregnant. Her obstetrician wants to do these lab studies to check her for both the routine obstetric blood work and a lipid profile:

(a) Complete automated blood count and the appropriate manual differential WBC count, hepatitis B, rubella antibody, syphilis test, qualitative, RBC antibody screen, blood typing ABO and Rh(D).

(b) Cholesterol serum total, lipoprotein, HDL cholesterol, triglycerides. Code the correct panels. _____

NAME _____

Medicine Section
Codes 90281–99607

The Medicine Section of CPT contains the codes for the many types of evaluation, therapeutic, and diagnostic procedures that physicians perform. Most are considered noninvasive, in contrast to surgical procedures. The following major types of services are listed: immunizations, infusions, and chemotherapy; psychiatric; dialysis; gastroenterology; ophthalmology; cardiovascular; vascular and pulmonary studies; allergy and clinical immunology; neurology and neuromuscular; physical rehabilitation; and special services.

CODING TIP

Injections

Injections and infusions of immune globulins, vaccines, toxoids, and other substances require two codes, one for administration and one for the particular vaccine or toxoid that is given. Chemotherapy and allergen immunotherapy, however, do not follow this guideline. The notes for each section should be observed. The AMA CPT website has the most recent new or revised vaccine product codes.

Provide the medicine codes for the following procedures. Include any necessary modifiers. In many cases, more than one code is required.

1. subcutaneous injection of human rabies immune globulin _____

2. human immune globulin, intramuscular administration _____

3. intramuscular injection of Lyme disease vaccine _____

4. immunization with hepatitis A and hepatitis B vaccine _____

5. psychoanalysis _____

6. biofeedback training _____

7. hemodialysis procedure and single physician evaluation _____

8. diagnostic gastroenterology procedure, unlisted _____

9. fluorescein angiography _____

10. speech Stenger test _____

11. coronary thrombolysis by intracoronary infusion _____

12. limited transcranial Doppler study of intracranial arteries _____

13. total vital capacity _____

14. prick tests with allergenic extracts for (a) house dust, (b) seasonal grasses, (c) trees, (d) common ragweed, and (e) goldenrod _____

15. rapid desensitization procedure, discontinued _____

16. Preparation of chemotherapy agent followed by arterial infusion, 3 hours _____

17. PUVA photochemotherapy _____

18. mandated occupational therapy reevaluation _____

19. IM injection of antibiotic _____

20. speech audiometry threshold test, one ear _____

Medicine Section *continued*

CODING TIP

Cardiac Catheterization

Cardiac catheterizations are the most commonly performed surgical procedure. Cardiac catheterization codes include the catheterization procedure itself, the injection procedure, and the imaging supervision and interpretation.

Be aware that cardiac catheterizations—the catheter insertion and the imaging supervision and interpretation services, not the injection procedure—each have a professional and a technical component. Unless the physician owns the laboratory, those codes are billed with the 26 modifier.

21. percutaneous transluminal pulmonary artery balloon angioplasty, three arteries _____

22. right heart catheterization in the hospital _____

23. catheter placement for coronary angiography, in physician-owned catheterization laboratory _____

24. unusually complicated and difficult combined right heart and retrograde left heart catheterization _____

25. indicator dilution studies with arterial and venous catheterization, subsequent, in the hospital _____

26. percutaneous retrograde left heart catheterization from the femoral artery; injection procedure during the catheterization for aortography; and imaging supervision, interpretation, and report for aortography—all in physician-owned cath laboratory

_____

27. right heart catheterization and retrograde left heart catheterization for congenital anomalies, in the hospital _____

28. catheter placement in venous coronary bypass graft for coronary angiography; injection procedure for opacification of venous bypass graft; and imaging supervision, interpretation, and report—all in physician-owned catheterization laboratory

_____

29. The patient is seen for chest pain and shortness of breath. After months of medical treatment, the patient has a stress test with abnormal findings, a cardiac catheterization is performed, and a blockage is found in one of the coronary arteries. The surgeon explains that the blockage can be treated by percutaneous angioplasty, referred to as a PTCA, which involves the placement of a catheter through the skin into the affected artery, deploying a balloon that will remove the blockage. Code for the PTCA.

_____

_____

30. A newborn is not breathing correctly, and a congenital defect is suspected. Her physician recommends transthoracic echocardiography to determine the cause of the problem, because he suspects a malformation in the aortic valve and mitral valve.

_____

_____

31. Due to what may be an adverse reaction to longtime use of an antidepressant, a patient requires EEG monitoring for 2 hours to determine the brain's electrical activity. Sensors are placed on the patient's head to measure and record that activity. The physician then reviews the information and reports on his findings.

_____

_____

32. After allergy testing, a patient is diagnosed with allergies to bee and hornet stings. She is sent to an allergy specialist who prepares the allergenic extract for injection into the patient. The specialist also provides the single injection of the two stinging insect venoms.

_____

_____

33. A mother brings her child in to the pediatrician's office for a well visit. She knows that today her child will be getting the vaccine for DTaP and MMR. Each vaccine will be given via a separate injection. Code for the injections.

_____

_____

Category II Codes

Codes 0001F–7025F

The Category II code set contains supplemental tracking codes to help collect data regarding services, such as prenatal care and tobacco use cessation counseling, that are known to contribute to good patient care. Having codes available reduces the amount of administrative time needed to gather these data from documentation.

The use of these codes is optional and does not affect reimbursement. These codes are, however, used for pay-for-performance reporting, such as the PQRI program under CMS, in which case a bonus payment may result. The codes are not required for correct coding and are not a substitute for Category I codes.

Category II codes have an alphabetical character as the fifth character following the four digits in the code. They are arranged according to the following categories:

- Modifiers
- Composite Codes
- Patient Management
- Patient History
- Physical Examination
- Diagnostic/Screening Processes or Results
- Therapeutic, Preventive, or Other Interventions
- Follow-up or Other Outcomes
- Patient Safety
- Structural Measures
- Nonmeasure Code Listing

CODING TIP

Category II Code Updates

Category II codes are released twice a year: January 1 and July 1. The current listing and its effective date are available on the Internet at www.ama-assn.org/go/CPT.

Provide the Category II codes for the following performance measures.

1. tobacco use cessation intervention, counseling _____

2. tobacco use, smoking, assessed _____

3. subsequent prenatal care visit _____

4. blood pressure, measured _____

5. postpartum care visit _____

Category III Codes

Codes 0019T–0339T

The Category III code set contains temporary codes for emerging technology, services, and procedures. If a Category III code is available for a new procedure, this code must be reported instead of a Category I unlisted code.

The codes in this section are not like CPT Category I codes, which require that the service/procedure be performed by many health care professionals in clinical practice in multiple locations and that FDA approval, as appropriate, has already been received. For these reasons, temporary codes for emerging technology, services, and procedures have been placed in a separate section of the CPT book. When a temporary service or procedure does meet these requirements, it is then listed as a Category I code in the appropriate section of the main text.

Category III codes have an alphabetical character as the fifth character following the four digits in the code.

CODING TIP

Category III Code Updates

Category III codes are released twice a year: January 1 and July 1. The current listing and its effective date are available on the Internet at www.ama-assn.org/go/CPT.

Provide the Category III codes for the following procedures.

1. measurement of holotranscobalamin _____

2. insertion of anterior segment aqueous drainage device, via an internal
   approach, into the suprachoroidal space _____

3. injection of platelet-rich plasma into the arm, with image guidance

   _____

4. replacing the thoracic unit of an artificial heart _____

5. breath test for heart transplant rejection _____

6. high-dose rate electronic brachytherapy, skin surface application,
   per faction _____

7. insertion of intracardiac ischemia monitoring system, with imaging
   supervision and interpretation, device only _____

8. insertion of anterior segment aqueous drainage device, without extraocular reservoir; internal approach _____

9. esophageal motility study with high-resolution esophageal pressure topography, interpretation and report _____

10. removal of subcutaneous implantable defibrillator pulse generator

_____

Health Care Common Procedure Coding System (HCPCS)

The Health Care Common Procedure Coding System (HCPCS) is used to report procedures and services not covered in CPT. HCPCS Level II is a HIPAA-mandated code set that is revised annually by CMS. New codes are effective January 1 of the year and must be used for services provided on or after that date.

Level II is made up of over two thousand five-digit alphanumeric codes for items that are not listed in CPT. Most of these items are supplies, materials, or injections that may be covered by Medicare. For example, a HCPCS code from the J series of the Level II codes is used for the material (drug) that is injected, rather than a CPT code. Some items are new services or procedures that are not covered in CPT. Level II codes start with a letter followed by four digits, such as J7620. Each section covers a related group of items:

Ambulance and other transport services and supplies
Medical and surgical supplies
Administrative, miscellaneous and investigational
Enteral and parenteral therapy
Outpatient PPS
Durable medical equipment
Procedures/professional services (temporary)
Alcohol and drug abuse treatment
Drugs administered other than oral method
Chemotherapy drugs
Durable medical equipment (DME) Medicare administrative contractors (MACs)
Orthotic procedures and services
Prosthetic procedures
Miscellaneous medical services
Pathology and laboratory services
Temporary codes
Diagnostic radiology services
Temporary national codes (non-Medicare)
National codes established for state Medicaid agencies
Vision services
Hearing services
Modifiers for HCPCS codes

The two-letter HCPCS modifiers are useful indicators of factors other than those covered by CPT modifiers. For example, there are HCPCS modifiers for each finger and each toe. The modifiers are to be used with both Level I and Level II codes.

HCPCS Level II codes and modifiers are available both from government sources and from many commercial publishers. Visit the CMS website for general HCPCS information at:

www.cms.gov/medhcpcsgeninfo/

CODING TIPS

Locating Correct HCPCS Codes

The steps for locating correct codes using HCPCS Level II codes and modifiers are similar to those for CPT codes. First, locate the main term in the index, and then check the section listings to verify accuracy. Similar format rules also apply. Descriptors before a semicolon are common; the entries after it provide unique endings to complete the procedure. Note, however, that unlike CPT, many codes are differentiated by quantities or dosages. Check also for the need for modifiers.

ABN Modifiers

HCPCS modifiers are used as CPT modifiers are used. For example, HCPCS modifiers distinguish between voluntary and required use of advanced beneficiary notices of noncoverage (ABNs):

GA Waiver of Liability Statement Issued as Required by Payer Policy, Individual Case

GX Notice of Liability Issued, Voluntary under Payer Policy

GK Reasonable and Necessary Item/Service Associated with GA or GZ Modifier

GY Item or Service Statutorily Excluded

GZ Item or Service Expected to Be Denied as Not Reasonable and Necessary

NAME _____

HCPCS Level II National Codes and Modifiers

Provide the HCPCS codes and modifiers for the following procedures.

1. standard wheelchair _____

2. adjustable semirigid cervical molded chin cup _____

3. WHFO without customized joint prefabricated item _____

4. 12-volt Utah battery and battery charger _____

5. cardiokymography _____

6. nonemergency BLS ambulance service _____

7. nasal cannula _____

8. occult blood test strips, for dialysis 100 _____

9. drainable ostomy pouch with attached barrier _____

10. Levine type stomach tube _____

11. dysphagia screening _____

12. hearing aid fitting _____

13. anterior chamber intraocular lens _____

14. scratch-resistant coating for a pair of glasses _____

15. static finger splint _____

16. 2 mg, dactinomycin _____

17. inhalation solution of beclomethasone, per milligram, DME administration, unit dose _____

18. isoetharine hydrochloride inhalation solution, DME administration, unit dose form, 1 mg _____

19. administration, influenza virus vaccine _____

20. individual smoking cessation counseling, 8 minutes _____

21. hemodialysis machine _____

22. total electric hospital bed with mattress _____

23. pickup folding walker, new _____

24. non-segmental home model, pneumatic compressor, rental _____

25. one gram of wound filler hydrocolloid dressing, dry form _____

For the following, supply the CPT (HCPCS Level I) code or codes, as well as HCPCS modifiers, if appropriate.

26. excision of 1.0-cm benign lesion from upper right eyelid _____

27. release of thenar muscle, left thumb _____

28. acute chiropractic manipulative treatment, one spinal region _____

29. anesthesia for closed procedure in hip joint personally performed by anesthesiologist _____

30. ligation of anomalous left anterior descending coronary artery

_____

31. hallux valgus correction, left foot, great toe _____

32. single determination, noninvasive pulse oximetry for oxygen saturation, technical component _____

33. extracapsular cataract extraction and insertion of IOL, performed in ambulatory surgical center _____

34. automated dip stick urinalysis, CLIA-waived test _____

35. closed treatment of acetabulum fracture with manipulation, right hip

_____

Coding Quiz: CPT and HCPCS

NAME _____

____ 1. A cardiovascular surgeon begins to perform a percutaneous transcatheter placement of an intracoronary stent, but stops the procedure because of the patient's respiratory distress. Select the correct code.

    ① 92921
    ② 92920
    ③ 92920 52
    ④ 92920 53

____ 2. A metal splinter was removed from the posterior segment of both eyes' ocular area using a magnet. Choose the correct code.

    ① 65260 52
    ② 65260 50
    ③ 65235
    ④ 65265

____ 3. A surgeon performs a diagnostic ERCP and a trocar bladder aspiration. Which codes are correct?

    ① 43260, 51101 22
    ② 43260, 51101 51
    ③ 43260, 51101 59
    ④ 43260, 51101 62

____ 4. A patient has an office encounter for removal of five skin tags on her hand. During the visit, she asks the physician to evaluate swelling and heat in her left knee. The physician performs an expanded history and examination with low medical decision making. What codes should be reported?

    ① 11200, 99214
    ② 11200, 99213 25
    ③ 11100, 99213 25
    ④ 11200, 99213 51

____ 5. Following surgery to repair a sliding inguinal hernia, the patient is turned over to his primary care physician for all follow-up care. Which is the correct code for that follow-up care?

    ① 49525 55
    ② 49525 25
    ③ 49525 77
    ④ 49525 24

_____ 6. What is the correct code for a home visit with an established patient that required a detailed history of what has occurred since the physician's previous visit, a detailed examination, and moderately complex medical decision making?

① 99243
② 99343
③ 99349
④ 99315

_____ 7. A patient is referred to a specialist, who performs an E/M service in the office and prepares a written report for the referring physician. From what code range is the correct code chosen?

① 99241–99245
② 99251–99255
③ 99281–99288
④ 99291–99292

_____ 8. Selecting a code from the range for emergency department services depends on

① whether the patient is new or established
② whether the patient is new or established, and what type of history is taken
③ the type of history, examination, and medical decision making performed
④ the type of history/examination performed and the amount of time spent

_____ 9. The physician is asked by the patient to perform a cardiovascular health risk assessment to evaluate his probability for heart disease. Which code is correct?

① 99401
② 99401 22
③ 99251
④ 96160

_____ 10. Modifier 47 is used for anesthesia services performed under difficult circumstances.

① True
② False

_____ 11. Which set of codes correctly describes the anesthesia services for insertion of a cardioverter-defibrillator via a transthoracic approach in a patient with severe systemic disease?

① 00534 P3
② 00560 P3
③ 00534 P4
④ 00560 P4

_____ **12.** The correct code for a postoperative visit for the purpose of documentation is

    ① 99070
    ② 99026
    ③ 99024
    ④ 99217

_____ **13.** A global surgery code for a diagnostic procedure includes follow-up care related only to recovery from the procedure itself, not for care of the patient's underlying condition.

    ① True
    ② False

_____ **14.** A patient's 3.9-cm benign lesion excision on the arm is followed by an intermediate repair involving a layered closure of 4.5 cm. Select the correct code(s).

    ① 11404
    ② 12002, 11424 51
    ③ 12002, 11404 51
    ④ 12032, 11404 51

_____ **15.** A surgeon applied a 75-sq cm skin substitute graft to the trunk. Select the correct code(s).

    ① 15272 × 3
    ② 15271
    ③ 15273
    ④ 15275

_____ **16.** A surgeon performed an excision of a chest wall tumor involving the ribs and then performed a mediastinal lymphadenectomy, followed by plastic reconstruction. Select the correct code(s).

    ① 19301, 19302 51
    ② 19260, 19272
    ③ 19272
    ④ 19301, 19272 51

_____ **17.** After initiating a regional Bier block, a surgeon performs a closed treatment of an ulnar shaft fracture; the surgeon monitored the patient and the block during the surgery. Select the correct code(s) for this service.

    ① 25530, 01820 47
    ② 25530 47
    ③ 25530
    ④ 01820, 25530

_____ **18.** Following the open treatment of a fractured big toe, the surgeon applies an ambulatory-type short leg cast. Choose the correct code(s).

   ① 28515
   ② 28525
   ③ 28505
   ④ 28505, 29425

_____ **19.** A patient had a previous operation 15 days ago to treat a dislocated ankle. Today, the same surgeon repairs the patient's flexor tendon on the other foot. What code should be reported for today's service?

   ① 28200 79
   ② 28200
   ③ 28200 58
   ④ 28200 51

_____ **20.** A physician removes a foreign body from a patient's nose during an office visit; local anesthesia was required. Should the anesthesia administration be reported for reimbursement?

   ① Yes
   ② No

_____ **21.** Diagnostic endoscopy is performed on the left nasal cavity. Select the correct code.

   ① 31237
   ② 31231 52
   ③ 31231 50
   ④ 31231

_____ **22.** Select the correct code(s) for a segmentectomy and bronchoplasty.

   ① 32484, 32501 51
   ② 32484, 32501
   ③ 32484, 31770 51
   ④ 32501

_____ **23.** A cardiologist performs a second pericardiocentesis and provides supervision/interpretation of the radiological procedures. Choose the correct code(s).

   ① 33010
   ② 33010 26
   ③ 33011, 76930
   ④ 33011, 76930 26

_____ **24.** Combined arterial and venous grafting for a coronary bypass is coded using the range 33517–33523.

   ① True
   ② False

_____ **25.** The repair of a ruptured aneurysm of the abdominal aorta is made extreme-
ly complicated by the patient's obesity; the procedure takes twice as long
as normally anticipated, which is appropriately documented in the operative report. Select the correct code.

① 35001

② 35082 59

③ 35082

④ 35082 22

_____ **26.** Following a diagnostic thoracoscopy and biopsy of the mediastinal space,
the surgeon performs a surgical thorascopy and excises a mediastinal
mass. Select the correct code(s).

① 32606, 32662 51

② 32606, 32662 59

③ 32662

④ 32601, 32606

_____ **27.** The correct reporting of a separate procedure that is not done as part of a
surgical package requires which of the following modifiers?

① 51

② 54

③ 59

④ 99

_____ **28.** The correct code for a laparoscopically aided esophagogastric fundo-
plasty is 43280. What is the code for the same procedure using an open
approach?

① 43289

② 43327

③ 43325

④ 49320

_____ **29.** A surgeon performs a modified radical mastectomy, including the axillary
lymph nodes, following an incisional breast biopsy, which results in a
finding of malignancy. Select the correct code(s) for these procedures.

① 19303, 19101

② 19303, 19101 51

③ 19307

④ 19303 52

_____ **30.** A cesarean delivery followed an attempted vaginal delivery. The mother's
previous children had been born with cesarean delivery. The physician han-
dled both the delivery and routine antepartum and postpartum care. Select
the correct code.

① 59618

② 59620

③ 59622

④ 59610

____ **31.** The surgeon created a twist drill hole for subdural puncture in order to implant a pressure recording device. Select the correct code(s).

    ① 61105, 61107 51
    ② 61105, 61107 59
    ③ 61105, 61107
    ④ 61107

____ **32.** Many radiology procedures have two parts:

    ① unlisted or guided.
    ② supervision or interpretation.
    ③ professional or technical.
    ④ complete or partial.

____ **33.** The correct code for an angiography of the internal mammary, including radiological supervision and interpretation, is

    ① 75756
    ② 75756 26
    ③ 75746
    ④ 75746 26

____ **34.** Select the correct code(s) for these laboratory tests: carbon dioxide, sodium, urea nitrogen, creatinine, chloride, calcium, glucose, and potassium.

    ① 82374, 84295, 84520, 82565, 82435, 82310, 82947, 84132
    ② 80051, 82310, 82565, 84520
    ③ 80053
    ④ 80048

____ **35.** A growth hormone stimulation panel and an aldosterone test are ordered. Choose the correct codes.

    ① 80428, 82088 51
    ② 80428, 82088
    ③ 80428, 82088 59
    ④ 80435, 82088

____ **36.** An intravenous injection of Gamunex 500 mg is administered to a Medicare patient. Choose the correct code(s).

    ① 90283, 96372
    ② 90281, 96374
    ③ J1561, 96374
    ④ J1561

_____ **37.** A cardiologist performed a percutaneous retrograde left heart cardiac catheterization for a left ventriculography. The cardiologist provided imaging supervision, interpretation, and report. Select the correct code(s).

① 93452, 93565
② 93458
③ 93452
④ 93453

_____ **38.** To study a patient's sleep disorder, a neurologist conducted an extended 4-hour monitoring of the patient's EEG. Choose the correct code.

① 95812
② 95813
③ 95813 22
④ 95819

_____ **39.** For a Medicare patient, which range of codes is used for prosthetic procedures?

① L5000–L9999
② M0064–M0301
③ J0120–J8999
④ A4206–A8004

_____ **40.** A Medicare patient is prescribed a wheelchair with detachable arms and leg rests. Which code is correct?

① E1050
② E1083
③ E1150
④ E1160

Part 3 Auditing Linkage and Compliance

U nder the regulations of HIPAA, providers are required to use multiple coding systems to code single episodes in order to satisfy the data needs for reimbursement, case mix analysis, practice profiling, research, and outcomes measurement. The illustration on the next page reviews the basic steps in the medical coding process and the code sets that are required for the various billing settings. As noted in Part 1, as of October 1, 2015, coding of diagnoses must be based on ICD-10-CM.

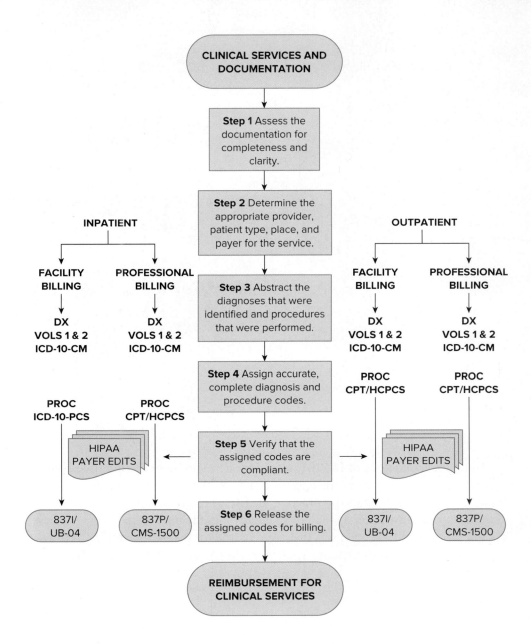

Facility (institutional) billing refers to charging payers and patients for the costs incurred by the hospital or other entity in the delivery of health care. *Professional billing,* on the other hand, refers to charging for the costs of providing physicians' or other professional providers' services, such as those of a surgeon, a nurse practitioner, or a CRNA. When the physician provides services, treatments, and procedures in the physician's office or other physician-owned setting, the physician's charges incorporate the cost of the "facility." When the physician performs professional work in the hospital, however, the physician is charging for the particular procedures, and the hospital is charging for the facility's part of the costs, such as:

- Room and board
- Medications
- Ancillary tests and procedures

- Equipment supplied/used during surgery or therapy
- The amount of time spent in an operating room, recovery room, or intensive care unit
- Administrative and patient care services

In the *inpatient* setting, for *facility billing,* the medical coder in the Health Information Management (HIM) department assigns both diagnosis and procedure codes based on the ICD-10-CM. The principal diagnosis (Pdx)—the condition established after study as the chief reason for the patient's admission—is listed first, followed by other, secondary diagnosis codes. The ICD-10-PCS (Procedure Coding System) is used along with the ICD-10-CM system. Both types of inpatient procedure codes result in reimbursement to the facility for all the services it provided.

In the *inpatient* setting, for *professional billing,* the medical coder who is employed by the physician practice assigns diagnosis codes based on ICD-10-CM and procedure codes based on CPT/HCPCS.

In the *outpatient* setting, for both *facility* and *professional billing,* the medical coder assigns diagnosis codes again based on ICD-10-CM. Procedures are coded using the CPT/HCPCS code set.

Code Linkage

On correct claims, each reported service is connected to a diagnosis that supports the necessity of the procedure to investigate or treat the patient's condition. This connection between the diagnostic and the procedural information, called *code linkage,* establishes the medical necessity—medical services' baseline—of the reported charges. Correct claims also comply with the many other requirements issued by government and private payers, such as those dealing with the place, frequency, and/or level of services or specific documentation.

To establish medical necessity, the payer must understand the patient's condition—how severe it is, or how it is emerging—and everything about signs, symptoms, or history that relates to the reason for care. These facts must be documented in the patient's medical record as well as in the codes.

Claims are denied due to lack of medical necessity when the reported services are not consistent with the symptoms or the diagnosis, or are not in keeping with generally accepted professional medical standards. Correctly linked codes that support medical necessity meet these conditions:

- The CPT procedure codes match the ICD-10-CM diagnosis codes.
- The procedures are not elective, experimental, or nonessential.
- The procedures are furnished at an appropriate level.

Medical necessity edits are established by each third-party payer. For example, Medicare carriers have their own rules for particular procedures and the diagnoses that must be linked for payment. Private payers may impose different edits.

Common Coding Errors

All codes must be currently correct and complete. Errors include:

- Truncated coding—diagnosis codes are not reported at the highest level of specificity available
- Using out-of-date codes

- Assumption coding—reporting items or services that are not actually documented, but that the coder assumes were performed
- Altering documentation after the services are reported
- Coding without proper documentation
- Reporting services provided by unlicensed or unqualified clinical personnel
- Failing to have all necessary documentation available at the time of coding
- Failing to satisfy the conditions of coverage for a particular service, such as the physician's direct supervision of a radiology technician's work
- Failing to comply with the unique billing requirements for a particular service, such as the rules for global surgical period coverage
- Reporting services that are not covered or that have limited coverage
- Using modifiers incorrectly, or not at all
- Upcoding—using a procedure code that provides a higher reimbursement rate than the code that actually reflects the service provided
- Unbundling—billing the parts of a bundled procedure as separate procedures

Coding Compliance

The *Medical Coding Workbook* is designed to build your skill in accurately linking diagnosis and procedure codes and correctly reporting them. Each set of exercises begins with a *Coding Tip* that explains an important rule concerning linkage and compliance. After completion of all the exercises in this part, you will know how to apply these guidelines:

- Verifying linkage
- Selecting the primary condition
- Reporting chronic or undiagnosed conditions
- Using Z and external cause codes under ICD-10-CM to form a clear picture of an encounter
- Avoiding unspecified diagnosis codes
- Reporting complications
- Reporting global procedures and laboratory panels
- Using correct code sets
- Following the *ICD-10-CM Official Guidelines for Coding and Reporting*

NAME _____

Section 1

CODING TIP

Verifying Linkage

Appropriately linked diagnosis and procedure codes pass the test of clinical consistency. When a condition has been diagnosed, other reported conditions and/or symptoms must be related to it, and treatments should be related to functional impairments and disabilities. For CPT evaluation and management (E/M) codes, the diagnosis code should support the level of the E/M code. For example, a diagnosis of dermatitis due to sunburn does not support the medical necessity of a comprehensive examination, even if the physician performs and documents all required components. For procedures, the diagnosis code should relate clinically to the procedure. Clinically, then, the overall coding of the case should be reasonable.

The following diagnosis and procedure codes have been reported. In each case, indicate whether the codes are correctly linked ("Y" for yes) or not correctly linked ("N" for no).

	ICD-10-CM	CPT	Linked?
1.	L55.0	99201	_____
2.	I21.09	99223	_____
3.	R31.9, R35.0, R10.84	50600	_____
4.	D23.10	67961	_____
5.	K56.0	27147	_____
6.	P08.22	99382	_____
7.	Q67.4	30520	_____
8.	E10.36	92012	_____
9.	S82.871A	27824	_____
10.	K66.0	56810	_____

Section 2

CODING TIP

Selecting the Primary Diagnosis

The primary diagnosis, or condition, is the most important reason for the care provided. It is reported first, if more than one condition is pertinent or treated. Additional codes are listed to describe all documented, current coexisting conditions that affect patient treatment or require treatment during the encounter. Coexisting conditions may be related to the primary diagnosis, or they may involve a separate illness that the physician diagnoses and treats during the encounter. Only the definitive condition or conditions that caused the encounter are coded. Symptoms that are integral to a diagnosis, such as stomach pain related to bowel obstruction, are not reported.

Some conditions require the assignment of two codes. A code may be needed for the disease's etiology and another for its manifestation, or typical signs or symptoms. Manifestation codes are never primary, even when the diagnostic statement is written in that order. In some cases, a combination code may cover both etiology and manifestation.

Provide the diagnosis codes for the following statements. If sufficient information is given, also provide the procedure code. List the ICD-10-CM codes in the correct order, followed by the CPT codes.

1. severe abdominal pain, nausea, and vomiting from acute pancreatitis

   _____

2. fatigue, enlarged spleen, and hereditary sideroblastic anemia

   _____

3. cerebellar ataxia and hepatitis in chronic episodic alcoholism

   _____

4. pneumonia due to parainfluenza virus; radiologic examination of chest, special views

   _____

5. generalized peritonitis and acute appendicitis; appendectomy for ruptured appendix

_____

6. direct ligation of esophageal varices due to portal hypertension

_____

7. patient complained of hematuria and pyuria; urinalysis by bacterial culture of urine by commercial kit confirms acute pyelonephritis due to *E. coli* infection

_____

8. physician performs cystourethroscopy with bilateral meatotomy to remove a foreign body in the genitourinary tract

_____

9. postsurgical malnutrition; a breath hydrogen test is performed

_____

10. due to dysmenorrhea and uterine endometriosis, physician performs a laparoscopic assisted vaginal hysterectomy, uterus less than 250 grams

_____

Section 3

CODING TIP

Reporting Chronic or Undiagnosed Conditions

A chronic condition—one that continues over a long period of time or recurs frequently—is reported each time the patient receives care for that condition. However, conditions that are no longer being treated or no longer exist are not reported, unless the documentation shows that a previous history is pertinent to the current condition. Some encounters cover both an acute and a chronic condition. If both the acute and the chronic illnesses are treated and each has a code, list the acute code first. Diagnoses are not always established at the first encounter. In this case, diagnosis codes that cover symptoms, signs, and ill-defined conditions are used. Inconclusive diagnoses, such as those preceded by "rule out," "suspected," or "probable," are not coded in the outpatient setting. Code only to the highest degree of certainty, listing the most definitive diagnosis first.

Provide the diagnosis codes for the following statements. If sufficient information is given, also provide the procedure code. List the ICD-10-CM codes in the correct order, followed by the CPT codes.

1. chronic and subacute arthropathy

   _____

2. encounter for chronic pleurisy with influenza

   _____

3. patient complains of blood in urine, frequent urination, and generalized abdominal pain; a tumor is suspected, and a diagnostic cystoscopy is scheduled

   _____

4. acute and chronic mesenteric lymphadenitis

   _____

5. vertigo; TIA suspected

   _____

6. generalized intraabdominal and pelvis swelling, probable malignant tumor

   _____

7. stereotactic needle core breast biopsy; finding of malignant primary tumor in upper-outer quadrant of left female breast

_____

8. routine 12-lead ECG with interpretation/report, abnormal finding

_____

9. patient with chronic and acute maxillary sinusitis undergoes surgical nasal/sinus endoscopy and maxillary antrostomy

_____

10. office consultation (comprehensive history and examination, moderately complex medical decision making) to evaluate complaints of nervousness, loss of sleep, and heat intolerance; diagnosis of thyrotoxicosis, factitia with storm; ruled out Graves' disease

_____

Section 4

CODING TIP

Using Z and External Cause Codes for a Clear Picture of an Encounter

Z codes, for factors influencing health status and contact with health services, and external cause codes, for external causes of injury and poisoning, are often required to provide a complete picture of the medical necessity for reported procedures. These codes may also help establish liability among payers, such as primary medical insurance and workers' compensation coverage.

Some Z codes, such as those for general medical examinations and screening tests, are used as primary diagnoses. Others, such as Z codes for a family or personal history of a disease, may not be used as primary; rather, they are listed as secondary codes. External cause codes are always secondary to the primary diagnosis, because their purpose is to describe a cause, not a condition or a reason for an encounter.

Remember that codes in categories T36–T65 are combination codes for the substances related to adverse effects, poisoning, toxic effects, and underdosing, as well as the external cause of these effects. When these combination codes are assigned, no additional external cause code is needed. The combination code is listed first, followed by the code for the manifestation.

Provide the diagnosis codes for the following statements. If sufficient information is given, also provide the procedure code. List the ICD-10-CM codes in the correct order, followed by the CPT codes.

1. single assay HIV-1 and HIV-2 screening test for AIDS; patient has no HIV-related symptoms

   _____

2. intramuscular injection of hepatitis B globulin

   _____

3. annual medical examination of a 49-year-old male who is a new patient

   _____

4. bilateral screening mammography of patient whose mother and sister were diagnosed with breast cancer

   _____

5. normal vaginal delivery, antepartum/postpartum care, delivery of healthy boy

   _____

6. patient is a house painter who fell from scaffolding on the job and required closed treatment and manipulation of a transverse fracture of the shaft of the humerus of his right arm

   _____

7. local treatment of first-degree burns on both lower legs of an adult after clothing was burned by a bonfire

   _____

8. therapeutic gastric intubation and aspiration by a physician to remove stomach contents

   _____

9. office encounter with an established patient (expanded history/ examination, low decision-making complexity) who has nausea and vomiting due to an adverse reaction to an antibiotic

   _____

10. surgical exploration of a complicated chest wound with penetration into thoracic cavity caused by shotgun accident

    _____

Section 5

CODING TIP

Avoiding Unspecified Diagnostic Codes

Unspecified diagnosis codes—usually those that end in 0 or 9 within a category—indicate that a particular body site was not documented, although classifications are available, or other information is not present. The lack of information causes selection of an unspecified code that may not prove medical necessity, because it is considered too vague to support the requirement for the procedure. When documentation is insufficient, often coders request more specific information.

For each of the following diagnostic statements, what information is missing that would permit the assignment of a specific ICD-10-CM code?

1. patient complains of abdominal pain

   _____

   _____

2. gastric or intestinal hemorrhage

   _____

   _____

3. chronic bronchitis

   _____

   _____

4. acute myocardial infarction, location specified

   _____

   _____

5. chronic suppurative otitis media

   _____

   _____

6. reaction to stress

   _____

   _____

7. diabetes mellitus

_____

_____

8. monocytic leukemia in remission

_____

_____

9. streptococcus infection

_____

_____

10. osteoarthrosis

_____

_____

Section 6

CODING TIP

Reporting Surgical Diagnoses and Complications

When surgery is performed and the preoperative diagnosis changes, the new postoperative diagnosis code is reported, rather than the preoperative code.

If complications arise during the procedure, the primary diagnosis is the first code reported. The complication is coded in addition, following the primary diagnosis. However, if the complications arise after the procedure is complete and require an additional procedure, the complication is the primary diagnosis for the later procedure.

Provide the diagnosis codes for the following statements. If sufficient information is given, also provide the procedure code. List the ICD-10-CM codes in the correct order, followed by the CPT codes.
Hint: **Some procedures require the use of a modifier.**

1. mechanical complication due to a breakdown of the cardiac electrode

   _____

2. accidental puncture of the spleen during surgery on the spleen

   _____

3. septicemia after repair of an open wound

   _____

4. vaccinia resulting from an immunization

   _____

5. complications arising after an incompatible blood transfusion

   _____

6. *Staphylococcus aureus* septicemia due to an indwelling urethral catheter

   _____

7. During a procedure to implant a patient-activated cardiac event recorder, a hemorrhage occurs.

   _____

8. Twelve hours following surgery for an acute myocardial infarction, the electrode of a cardiac pacemaker fails, requiring additional surgery.

_____

9. Following removal of a 2.5-cm tumor from the uterus of a patient, the pathology report indicates that it is malignant.

_____

10. A laparoscopic cholecystectomy is performed for a patient with acute cholecystitis; during the procedure, the patient has cardiac arrest, and after reviving the patient with CPR, the surgeon terminates the procedure.

_____

NAME _____

Section 7

Provide both the diagnostic and procedure codes for the following statements.

1. During an annual physical examination of a 62-year-old female established patient with a family history of kidney disease, the physician orders a comprehensive metabolic panel and a renal function panel.

   _____

2. Patient has bloody stool; physician performs a diagnostic sigmoidoscopy followed by removal of a foreign body.

   _____

3. Patient has a transverse fracture of the left tibial shaft; physician performs a closed treatment and applies an ambulatory short leg cast.

   _____

4. Following a biopsy, two benign sebaceous cystic skin lesions are excised—a 4.2-cm lesion from the hand of the patient and a 3.3-cm lesion from the patient's back; surgeon administered local anesthesia.

   _____

5. Patient has suffered an open fracture of multiple sites of her lower jaw bone when the car in which she was a passenger hit the highway divider; surgeon performs an open treatment that requires multiple approaches, including internal fixation, interdental fixation, and wiring of dentures.

   _____

6. Physician performs an endoscopically aided diagnostic bronchoscopy and a transbronchial lung biopsy under fluoroscopic guidance for a patient with pneumonia due to adenovirus.

   _____

7. Physician orders laboratory tests of total serum cholesterol, direct measurement of HDL cholesterol, and triglycerides for a patient with essential hypertension.

   _____

8. Elderly patient has been diagnosed with a cortical age-related cataract in the left eye; surgeon performs a one-stage extracapsular cataract removal with iridectomy, use of viscoelastic agents, and subconjunctival injections, and then inserts an intraocular lens prosthesis.

   _____

9. Patient has been diagnosed with carcinoma in situ of the prostate; surgeon performs a complete transurethral electrosurgical resection of the prostate; the procedure includes a vasectomy, meatotomy, cystourethroscopy, urethral calibration, and internal urethrotomy; control of postoperative bleeding is also required.

   _____

10. After a comprehensive ophthalmological examination of a new Medicare patient and a finding of an age-related nuclear cataract of the left eye, the corneal lens is replaced, and supplying the bifocal gas permeable contact lens is also reported.

   _____

Section 8

CODING TIPS

ICD-10-PCS

The change to ICD-10-PCS (Procedure Coding System) for inpatient procedural reporting for hospitals and payers expands the code set from 4,000 codes to more than 87,000 codes. ICD-10-PCS replaced ICD-9-CM Volume 3 and is mandated for facility reporting of hospital inpatient procedures.

Code Set Structure

ICD-10-PCS has a multiaxial code structure. This term means that a table format is used to present options for building a code. An axis is a column or row in a table; columns are vertical, while rows are horizontal. The coder picks the correct values from one of the rows in a table to build a code for each procedure. This approach provides a unique code for every substantially different procedure and allows new procedures to be easily incorporated as new codes.

   The code set is contained both online and in a printed reference. It is updated annually. The Code Tables, the main part of the code set, begin with an index to assist in locating common procedures. Then procedures are divided into 16 sections that identify the general type of procedure, such as medical and surgical, obstetrics, or imaging. The first character of the procedure code always specifies the section:

Sections	
0	Medical and Surgical
1	Obstetrics
2	Placement
3	Administration
4	Measurement and Monitoring
5	Extracorporeal Assistance and Performance
6	Extracorporeal Therapies
7	Osteopathic
8	Other Procedures
9	Chiropractic
B	Imaging
C	Nuclear Medicine
D	Radiation Oncology
F	Physical Rehabilitation and Diagnostic Audiology
G	Mental Health
H	Substance Abuse Treatment

Each section is made up of a series of tables, with columns and rows for valid combinations of codes.

ICD-10-PCS follows a logical, consistent structure. Codes in ICD-10-PCS are built using individual letters and numbers, called "values," selected in sequence to occupy the seven spaces of the code, called "characters."

Characters: All codes in ICD-10-PCS are seven characters long. Each character in the seven-character code represents an aspect of the procedure.

For example, in the medical/surgical section, the characters mean the following:

Character 1 = Section

Character 2 = Body System

Character 3 = Root Operation

Character 4 = Body Part

Character 5 = Approach

Character 6 = Device

Character 7 = Qualifier

Values: One of 34 possible values can be assigned to each character in a code: the numbers 0–9 and the alphabet (except I and O, because they are easily confused with the numbers 1 and 0). A finished code looks like the example below.

02103D4

This code is built by choosing a specific value for each of the seven characters. The columns specify the allowable values for characters 4–7, and the rows specify the valid combinations of values. As an example, review this table for the medical and surgical root operation dilation of the heart and great vessels body system (027):

0: Medical and Surgical
2: Heart and Great Vessels
7: Dilation: Expanding an orifice or the lumen of a tubular body part

Body Part Character 4	Approach Character 5	Device Character 6	Qualifier Character 7
0 Coronary Artery, One Site	**0** Open	**4** Intraluminal Device, Drug-eluting	**6** Bifurcation
1 Coronary Artery, Two Sites	**3** Percutaneous	**D** Intraluminal Device **T** Radioactive Intraluminal Device	**Z** No Qualifier
2 Coronary Artery, Three Sites **3** Coronary Artery, Four or More Sites	**4** Percutaneous Endoscopic	**Z** No Device	

Because the definition of each character is a function of its physical position in the code, the same value placed in a different position in the code means something different. For example, the value 0 in the first character means something different from 0 in the second character or 0 in the third character. Details about the procedure performed and values for each character specifying the section, body system, root operation, body part, approach, device, and qualifier are assigned.

These codes are examples of building from the above table:

027004Z	Dilation of Coronary Artery, One Site with Drug-eluting Intraluminal Device, Open Approach
02700DZ	Dilation of Coronary Artery, One Site with Intraluminal Device, Open Approach
02700ZZ	Dilation, Coronary Artery, One Site, Open Approach
027034Z	Dilation, Coronary Artery, One Site with Drug-eluting Intraluminal Device, Percutaneous Approach

Coding Procedure and Resources

The index of the ICD-10-PCS Code Tables lists the common procedures. Each entry shows the first three or four characters of the code, which point to the correct table to use to build the code.

After finding the index entry, the coder turns to the correct table, which has those digits in its table header, and selects values from the columns to assign values for the fourth, fifth, sixth, and seventh characters. All the characters must come from the same row (the left-to-right axis). After the coder is familiar with the table structure, it is not required to first consult the index to build an ICD-10-PCS code.

Coders use both the Code Tables/Index and the ICD-10-PCS Reference Manual, which contains explanatory and reference material. Also available on the CMS website are Coding Guidelines and GEMs (General Equivalent Mappings) that relate new to old codes.

A. Provide the diagnostic codes for the following statements.

1. Patient presents to the hospital with nausea and vomiting 4 hours after receiving chemotherapy for acute lymphocytic leukemia. She is readmitted for IV fluids and antiemetics. It is determined the nausea and vomiting are due to the chemotherapy.

   Principal/Other Diagnoses _____

2. Patient presents to the emergency room complaining of dizziness and head-ache postoperative day 6 from a primary cesarean section. Blood pressure upon presentation is 178/92. She is admitted for observation and monitoring for eclampsia.

   Principal/Other Diagnoses _____

3. Patient was recently hospitalized for pneumonia. He was discharged on moxi-floxacin. Two days following discharge, he reported onset of diarrhea. The patient was admitted and *Clostridium difficile* antigen came back positive. He also had evidence of acute renal failure due to dehydration. He was treated with Flagyl p.o. and vigorous hydration and continued treatment for pneumonia.

   Principal/Other Diagnoses _____

4. The patient is a newborn baby delivered by cesarean section at 35 weeks for intolerance of labor. Birth weight is 1730 grams. The baby is diagnosed with apnea of prematurity and transient thrombocytopenia.

Principal/Other Diagnoses _____

5. Patient is a 21-month-old male with 1-week history of fever and increased work of breathing. He is admitted, and DFA comes back positive for RSV bronchiolitis. He is given supplemental oxygen and weaned to room air as tolerated. He is also treated for hyponatremia due to dehydration.

Principal/Other Diagnoses _____

6. This 25-year-old female patient is admitted to the hospital for laparoscopic gastric bypass for morbid obesity. She has a body mass index of 53. She also presents with hypertension, hyperlipidemia, and diabetes without complications.

Principal/Other Diagnoses _____

7. Male patient presents to the emergency room with epistaxis. He thinks he may have accidently taken an extra dose of Coumadin which he takes for persistent atrial fibrillation. Lab results show an abnormal coagulation profile. He is admitted for observation and Coumadin is held. Epistaxis resolves, and he is discharged home in stable condition on regular dose of Coumadin.

Principal/Other Diagnoses _____

8. The patient is admitted to the hospital in acute respiratory failure. She is intubated and maintained on mechanical ventilation. She has a history of congestive heart failure for which she receives Lasix. Patient is diagnosed with acute respiratory failure with hypercapnia due to acute systolic heart failure.

Principal/Other Diagnoses _____

9. Mr. Cook presents to the emergency room with 3 days of nausea and vomiting. He is admitted in acute renal failure due to dehydration. He also has a history of end stage renal disease due to diabetic nephropathy and hypertension for which he receives hemodialysis. Acute renal failure resolves with IV hydration. He also receives regularly scheduled hemodialysis while inpatient. Nausea and vomiting are determined due to viral gastroenteritis which resolves on its own.

Principal/Other Diagnoses _____

10. The patient is admitted with chest pain and shortness of breath. Cardiac risk factors include hypertension and hyperlipidemia. The patient is also a smoker. Cardiac catherization shows coronary atherosclerosis. The patient is treated with coronary angioplasty and stent for unstable angina.

Principal/Other Diagnoses _____

B. Code the following inpatient cases, providing both diagnosis and procedure codes as assigned.

1. HISTORY OF PRESENT ILLNESS: The patient is a pleasant 48-year-old female with past medical history significant for hypertension, mild, intermittent asthma, and L3–L4 herniated nucleus pulposus. The patient continued to have low back pain as well as right lower extremity radiculopathy and has failed conservative treatment, therefore presents now for further surgical intervention. Current medications are Cardizem and Maxzide inhaler as needed for asthma exacerbation. There are no known allergies.

   HOSPITAL COURSE: Following informed consent including risks and benefits of surgical intervention as well as risk stratification by the patient's primary care physician, the patient was brought to the Operating Room, at which time she underwent an L3–L4 lumbar diskectomy. The patient tolerated the procedure well with no complications. The patient during the hospital stay continued to be monitored closely. On postoperative day 1, the patient noted to be hemodynamically and clinically stable and therefore disposition planning was initiated. At the time of dictation, the patient is tolerating a regular p.o. diet, is transitioning to oral pain medication, and will be seen today by Physical Therapy for clearance to home.

   FINAL DIAGNOSIS: L3–L4 Herniated nucleus pulposus

   PRINCIPAL DIAGNOSIS and CODE(S) _____

   OTHER DIAGNOSES and CODE(S) _____

   PROCEDURE CODE(S) _____

2. HISTORY OF PRESENT ILLNESS: This is a 60-year-old male who was diagnosed with a pituitary adenoma. Past medical history of hypertension and hyperlipidemia. He has no known drug allergies. The patient was consented and scheduled for surgery.

   HOSPITAL COURSE: The patient was admitted for percutaneous endoscopic transsphenoidal transseptal pituitary tumor resection. The patient remained in the Neurosurgical ICU overnight and remained stable overnight. ENT Team followed him throughout his stay. On postoperative day 1, he was transferred to the regular Neurosurgery Floor where he remained in stable condition and was seen by both Physical Therapy and Occupational Therapy Team. On postoperative day 2, the patient was noted to have some swelling in his lips and his left eye, and the Dermatology Team was consulted for possible allergic reaction. They felt that it was not an allergic resection, but it was impetigo. He was placed on doxycycline for a total of 10 days. The patient was discharged home in stable condition.

   FINAL DIAGNOSIS: Pituitary adenoma

   PRINCIPAL DIAGNOSIS and CODE(S) _____

   OTHER DIAGNOSES and CODE(S) _____

   PROCEDURE CODE(S) _____

3. **HISTORY OF PRESENT ILLNESS:** This is a 23-year-old male who initially presented 6 months ago complaining of double vision, rapidly enlarging right inguinal mass, jaw pain, numb chin, and inability to close the left eye. He had a biopsy of one of his lymph nodes, which was consistent with Burkitt lymphoma. CSF fluid and bone marrow biopsy were both positive for lymphoma. He has since received three cycles of chemotherapy. Most recently, the patient developed some left testicular/groin pain. CT of the abdomen and pelvis showed a 1.4-mm calculus in the left kidney, and this was believed to be the cause of the pain. The patient presents now for cycle 4 of chemotherapy. Surgical history is noncontributory, and he has no known allergies.

HOSPITAL COURSE: This is a 23-year-old male with stage IV Burkitt lymphoma admitted for cycle 4 of chemotherapy. He tolerated the regimen without any complications. The patient's urine was drained during this admission; however, he did not pass any stone despite aggressive hydration that he received with IV chemotherapy. He was discharged home in stable condition.

FINAL DIAGNOSIS: Burkitt lymphoma

PRINCIPAL DIAGNOSIS and CODE(S) _____

OTHER DIAGNOSES and CODE(S) _____

PROCEDURE CODE(S) _____

4. **HISTORY OF PRESENT ILLNESS:** The patient is an 81-year-old gentleman, who presents to the Emergency Room from an ECF with a fever of 103. He was complaining of abdominal pain and nausea. His past medical history includes metastatic prostate cancer status post prostatectomy with bony metastatic disease to the lumbar spine, chronic renal insufficiency, with a baseline creatinine of 1.5 to 1.7, history of coronary artery disease, status post pacemaker, hypertension, chronic anemia, and recurrent, mild depression. Current medications are Imdur and amlodipine. He is allergic to penicillin.

HOSPITAL COURSE: Fever and leukocytosis: The patient was started on vancomycin and Bactrim for a nosocomial pneumonia. Cultures revealed no growth on his blood cultures × 2 sets, and his urine culture was ultimately mixed flora. The patient defervesced and subsequently had improvement on the vancomycin and the Bactrim.

The vancomycin was discontinued, and the patient was watched on Bactrim alone for 2 days during which time he did not become febrile and additionally clinically remained unchanged.

Acute renal failure: The patient's renal function appeared to have bumped to 2.0 from his baseline of 1.5 to 1.7. He was given IV fluids with subsequent improvement back down to his baseline.

Metastatic prostate cancer: His pain was under fair control; he did respond quite well to the Toradol. However, this was not given on a long-term basis given his underlying chronic kidney disease.

Constipation: The patient appears to have had a history of nausea preventing him from having a good appetite and eating. He reported that he had been having frequent stool that was reported by the exam as well as an abdominal x-ray which showed stool in the colon. He was started on an aggressive bowel regimen with lactulose and Colace. With passing of his bowel movement, the patient's nausea reportedly did improve. The patient also had a CAT scan of his brain to rule out metastasis as a secondary cause for the nausea. The CT was unremarkable.

FINAL DIAGNOSIS: Nosocomial pneumonia

PRINCIPAL DIAGNOSIS and CODE(S) _____

OTHER DIAGNOSES and CODE(S) _____

PROCEDURE CODE(S) _____

5. HISTORY OF PRESENT ILLNESS: This patient is a 29-year-old with intrauterine pregnancy at 38 weeks. The patient was admitted to the hospital stating that she had not had any fetal movement for over 24 hours. The patient was told to come to the hospital immediately for evaluation.

HOSPITAL COURSE: On arrival, the patient was placed on the monitor, was noted to have a deceleration to approximately 90 beats per minute with a recovery followed shortly thereafter by a 2nd deceleration to 60 for another 2 minutes, heart rate then stabilized at 150 for several minutes and deceleration reoccurred. The patient was informed immediately that a low cervical cesarean section was necessary. The patient was quickly taken to the Operating Room, and spinal anesthesia was placed without difficulty. Once the heart rate was noted to be approximately 150, the patient was then prepped and draped and underwent a cesarean section. The postoperative course was unremarkable. She was discharged to home on postoperative day 4. The patient is to follow up in 6 weeks.

FINAL DIAGNOSIS: Intrauterine pregnancy with decreased fetal movement

PRINCIPAL DIAGNOSIS and CODE(S) _____

OTHER DIAGNOSES and CODE(S) _____

PROCEDURE CODE(S) _____

6. HISTORY OF PRESENT ILLNESS: The patient is a 75-year-old female who presents for postmenopausal vaginal bleeding. Endometrial biopsy is consistent with endometrial adenocarcinoma. Past medical history of polymyalgia rheumatica, hypertension, thyroid nodules, mild and recurrent depression, as well as a right knee replacement. Current medications are Prednisone 5, Hyzaar, Synthroid, and Lexapro.

PHYSICAL EXAMINATION: Vitals are within normal limits. The patient is in no apparent distress. Chest is clear. Heart is regular. Abdomen is soft and benign. Pelvic shows normal vulva, induration of the anterior vaginal wall, suburethral fissures in the small 14-week size nontender uterus. Adnexa are nontender and nonpalpable. Rectal is confirmatory.

HOSPITAL COURSE: The patient was admitted for surgical management of endometrial adenocarcinoma. She underwent laparoscopic vaginal hysterectomy, bilateral salpingo-oophorectomy, pelvic lymph node dissection, and a cystoscopy. Postoperatively, the patient did well. She quickly ambulated and tolerated regular diet and p.o. pain medications. She was given 1 dose of stress dose Solu-Cortef given her history of polymyalgia rheumatica with prednisone use. She was discharged to home on postoperative day 1 in good condition.

FINAL DIAGNOSIS: Endometrial adenocarcinoma

PRINCIPAL DIAGNOSIS and CODE(S) _____

OTHER DIAGNOSES and CODE(S) _____

PROCEDURE CODE(S) _____

7. HISTORY OF PRESENT ILLNESS: This is an 87-year-old woman who presents with a dislodged jejunostomy tube for replacement. The tube was nonfunctioning and missing parts on arrival and draining clear fluid. Therefore, a clamp was placed. Interventional Radiology was consulted and the patient was scheduled for a late afternoon or evening procedure. She was admitted for monitoring for that procedure. Past medical history is significant for diabetes and deep vein thrombosis on lower extremities. She also has a history of a stage IV sacral decubitus ulcer. She has a history of multiple sclerosis with paraplegia, and she is not ambulatory. History of recurrent UTIs, right above knee amputation secondary to nonhealing ulcer and hypertension. She also has hypothyroidism following thyroidectomy and a history of dementia. Current medications consist of Aricept, levothyroxine, a cranberry tablet per J-tube daily, Lopressor, and Coumadin. She is on tube feeds of Jevity every 4 hours.

PHYSICAL EXAMINATION: On admission to the floor, she was afebrile at 97.7, her heart rate was 93, blood pressure 140/78, respiratory rate 18, and saturating 97% on 2 L nasal canula. In general, she is awake and oriented to self. Speaks clearly and appropriately.

HEENT exam: Normocephalic and atraumatic. Her pupils 1 mm and minimally reactive to light. Extraocular movements were intact. Her oropharynx looked clear. Her mucous membranes were moist. Her neck showed no lymphadenopathy. It was supple. Full range of motion. Her right eye had a subconjunctival hemorrhage. Cardiac exam was regular rate and rhythm. Pulmonary with clear auscultation anteriorly. Abdomen was soft, nontender, and nondistended. She had good bowel sounds, and the J-tube site was clean, dry, and intact with the tube that was cut and clamped. She has intact sensation in her right AKA. As far as her skin, showed a stage IV 4 × 2 cm sacral decubitus ulcer that was packed and it had clean margins.

HOSPITAL COURSE: Interventional Radiology was notified that she was scheduled for a placement, which was performed in the evening. We held her Coumadin for 1 dose, but this should be restarted immediately. We had to hold her medications because her J-tube was not functioning, but those were restarted subsequently. Her fingersticks were checked every

6 hours, and she was given normal saline at 75 cc/h continuously. For her stage IV decubitus ulcer, we did dry-to-dry dressing with Nu Gauze packing and Xeroform and ordered an Eclipse bed for her. She was full code during this hospitalization, and she did very well and had an uneventful J-tube placement via previous artificial opening. Her tube feeds were restarted, Jevity 1.5 at a goal of 50 cc/h, and her outpatient medications are unchanged.

FINAL DIAGNOSIS: Jejunostomy tube displacement

PRINCIPAL DIAGNOSIS and CODE(S) _____

OTHER DIAGNOSES and CODE(S) _____

PROCEDURE CODE(S) _____

8. HISTORY OF PRESENT ILLNESS: The patient is an 88-year-old female presenting with an altered mental status. The patient complains of some burning with urination, has been urinating more frequently, and has also decreased appetite. She denies any fevers, night sweats, or chills. She also denies any headache, neck pain, or blurry vision. In the Emergency Department, she was febrile at a temperature of 100.1, pulse of 107, respirations 18, blood pressure 150/79, and saturating 98% on room air. Her past medical history is significant for chronic atrial fibrillation with rate control on Coumadin, congestive heart failure, diastolic dysfunction, mild mitral regurgitation. Other history includes diabetes type 2, hypertension, Paget's disease, asthma, and dyslipidemia. Current medications include lisinopril, Lasix, diltiazem, digoxin, warfarin, glipizide, simvastatin, and Protonix. She is allergic to penicillin.

HOSPITAL COURSE: The patient presented to the Emergency Room with altered mental status, likely in the context of urinary tract infection, and received ceftriaxone. She was also given gentle IV hydration. Blood cultures were obtained as well as urinary culture. Urinary culture grew out Klebsiella also consistent with her urinalysis findings being nitrite negative; therefore, she was continued on ceftriaxone for 3 days IV while in-house and will be discharged on 3 additional days of ciprofloxacin 500 mg p.o. b.i.d. Her blood cultures failed to elaborate any evidence of bacteremia. Rate control was achieved parenterally with metoprolol 5 mg IV q.6 hours with her ventricular response rate remaining in the 70 to 80 range. We held her Coumadin overnight. Once she was able to take p.o., we were able to restart her Coumadin as well as the rest of her cardiac medications including lisinopril and Cardizem. Her hyponatremia at the time of admission was initially thought to be secondary to hypovolemic hyponatremia. She was gently rehydrated with isotonic saline, and her sodium improved at the time of discharge. Additionally, for her diabetes, she was covered with sliding scale insulin while n.p.o., and then restarted on her oral hypoglycemics. The remainder of her medical issues remained stable.

FINAL DIAGNOSIS: Klebsiella urinary tract infection

PRINCIPAL DIAGNOSIS and CODE(S) _____

OTHER DIAGNOSES and CODE(S) _____

PROCEDURE CODE(S) _____

9. HISTORY OF PRESENT ILLNESS: This is a 64-year-old gentleman status post-fall from a roof approximately 15 feet with positive loss of consciousness. The patient was admitted for management of a right frontal subdural hematoma. The past medical history is significant for obesity, hypertension, diabetes mellitus, and hyperlipidemia. Current medications are Actos, glimepiride, lisinopril, aspirin, and simvastatin. There are no known drug allergies.

HOSPITAL COURSE: The patient was admitted to the ICU setting with neurosurgery consult. CT brain was performed. CT brain showed a small subdural hematoma along the medial aspect of the right frontal lobe. Cervical spine showed no acute traumatic injury. The patient had a repeat head CT, which showed the small extraaxial hematoma was stable. The patient was transferred out of the ICU setting to the floor. The patient had a right ankle fracture, managed by Orthopedics. Splint was applied. Orthopedics had recommended pain management, elevation of the right lower extremity, nonweightbearing and splint for 4 to 6 weeks. The patient had a right renal subcapsular hematoma. The patient did have some hypertension during his hospital stay as well as some hyperglycemia. The patient was placed on his home medications and Lopressor had been increased. The patient had been placed back on his home medication of lisinopril. Hypertension improved with these medications. The patient was placed back on glimepiride; the patient had a tight sliding scale regimen, and blood sugars had improved with this. The pain has been well controlled with oral pain medication.

FINAL DIAGNOSIS: Right frontal subdural hematoma, fracture distal tibia/fibula, renal subcapsular hematoma

PRINCIPAL DIAGNOSIS and CODE(S) _____

OTHER DIAGNOSES and CODE(S) _____

PROCEDURE CODE(S) _____

10. HISTORY OF PRESENT ILLNESS: The patient is an 83-year-old female who noticed slurring of her speech and an inability to remember people around her. She felt that she had indications of a slight stroke. The patient has had a previous stroke where she feels that she is weak on her right side but feels that these symptoms worsened. The patient's family described that initially the patient was disoriented and did not seem to be following instructions well but that had cleared up and she seems to be having a hard time getting words out. Her past medical history is significant for old MCA stroke with residual dysphasia and right hemiparesis, hypertension, chronic anemia, and cardiac pacemaker. Current medications include Toprol, Norvasc, and Plavix. The patient has no allergies.

PHYSICAL EXAMINATION: On initial physical exam, her vital signs were heart rate 61, blood pressure 164/75, respiratory rate 22, her oxygen saturation was 100% on room air. In general, she was lying in her bed in no apparent distress. HEENT and Neck Exam: Clear to auscultation. No carotid artery bruits. Cardiovascular: Regular rate and rhythm. No murmurs, rubs, or gallops. Lungs were clear to auscultation bilaterally. Abdominal exam was nontender, nondistended with good bowel sounds. Extremities had no edema. Neurological Exam: Her mental status was alert. She was cooperative. She perseverated. Her repetition was intact. She was able to read 2 words but perseverated on the words. She was not following commands. She was not alert and oriented. Cranial Nerves: Pupils were equal, round, and reactive to light. Extraocular movements were grossly intact. She had a right lower facial droop. Sensation was not tested and hearing was grossly intact. Her motor exam, on the right upper extremity, was 0/5. She was able to lift her right lower extremity minimally from the bed and she had 5/5 strength in her left upper extremity and left lower extremity. At her sensory exam, she grimaced to nail bed pressure in all four extremities. Coordination and gait were not tested.

HOSPITAL COURSE: The patient is status post-left MCA stroke as diagnosed by head CT with worsening aphasia. She was started on aspirin 325 mg daily p.r.n. She had physical therapy for gait training and occupational therapy for dressing technique and was evaluated for aphasia by the speech therapist who recommended home speech therapy at 3 times per week. The patient was found to have greater than 1000 Escherichia coli sent on urinalysis, confirming a urinary tract infection. She was started on Bactrim one double strength tablet q.12 hours.

FINAL DIAGNOSIS: New left MCA stroke with aphasia _____

PRINCIPAL DIAGNOSIS and CODE(S) _____

OTHER DIAGNOSES and CODE(S) _____

PROCEDURE CODE(S) _____

Coding Quiz: ICD-10-CM Auditing Linkage and Compliance

NAME _____

____ **1.** Which of the following is *not* required for correctly linked codes?

① The diagnosis and procedure codes present a logical clinical relationship.
② The diagnosis and procedures codes are from the same data set.
③ The procedures are necessary and effective and are not elective or experimental.
④ The treatment is provided at an appropriate level for the presenting problem.

____ **2.** In the diagnostic statement "eye dryness and irritation from insufficient tear production," the primary diagnosis is

① eye dryness
② eye irritation
③ tear production
④ insufficient tear production

____ **3.** The patient presents with transient infiltrations of the lungs by eosinophilia, resulting in cough, fever, and dyspnea. Select the correct diagnosis code(s).

① R05, R06.00
② R06.01, R05
③ J82
④ R50.9, R05, R06.0

____ **4.** Computed tomography without contrast is performed on the maxillofacial area for a patient with chronic sinusitis. Select the correct diagnosis and procedure codes.

① J32, 70486
② J32.4, 70486
③ J32.9, 70486
④ J32.0, 70486

____ **5.** An inconclusive diagnosis is indicated by terms such as

① rule out, suspected, probable
② finding, result, report
③ malignant, benign, in situ
④ adverse effect, poisoning, unspecified

_____ 6. Following catheterization and introduction of contrast material, a hysterosono-graphic study with radiological supervision and interpretation is conducted for a patient with postmenopausal bleeding and suspected endometrial carcinoma. Select the correct diagnosis and procedure codes.

① D49.59, 58350, 76831
② C54.1, 58340, 76831 26
③ N95.0, 58340, 76831 26
④ N95.0, C54.1, 58340, 76831

_____ 7. A biopsy of a dark growth on the back of a patient's hand reported a finding of a 0.9-cm malignant lesion, which was excised under local anesthesia. Select the correct diagnosis and procedure codes.

① C43.60, 17261 47
② C49.5, 17261
③ C76.40, 11621
④ C44.601, 11621

_____ 8. Select the correct codes for an annual physical examination of a 4-year-old established patient.

① Z00.00, 99392
② Z00.129, 99392
③ Z00.121, 99382
④ Z00.8, 99401

_____ 9. Following exposure to possible rabies from a dog bite, the patient is inoc-ulated intramuscularly with a rabies vaccine. Choose the correct codes.

① Z23, W54.0XXA, 90675, 90471
② W54.0XXA, Z20.3, 90675, 90471
③ Z20.3, W54.0XXA, 90675, 90471
④ Z20.3, W54.0XXA, 90675, 90471

_____ 10. Both Z codes and external cause codes may be primary or secondary, depending on the circumstances involved.

① True
② False

_____ 11. Select the correct diagnosis code for the following statement: "The patient suffers from atherosclerotic heart disease caused by plaque deposits in a grafted internal mammary artery. The patient underwent this arterial bypass graft procedure 4 months ago."

① I25.3
② I25.10
③ I25.810
④ I25.9

_____ **12.** When the physician owns the equipment and provides the supplies and technical service when providing radiology procedures, the 26 modifier is not appropriate.

① True
② False

_____ **13.** After introduction of anesthesia for an intracranial vascular procedure, the patient suddenly went into respiratory distress and the procedure was terminated. What is the correct code for the anesthesia service?

① 00216 53
② 00216
③ 00210 53
④ 61105 53

_____ **14.** In most cases, a biopsy of a site performed with a definitive procedure such as an excision or surgical removal of an organ is not coded.

① True
② False

_____ **15.** A patient had a total abdominal hysterectomy 35 days ago and has had increasing pain in the area of the incision. The surgeon performs a diagnostic laparoscopy and, finding adhesions, performs a surgical lysis. Select the correct codes.

① N73.6, 58200
② N99.4, 58660
③ N73.6, 58660 78
④ N99.4, 58660 78

_____ **16.** As part of a routine physical examination of a 70-year-old female Medicare patient who sees the doctor every year, the primary care physician orders tests sent to an outside laboratory for total serum cholesterol, HDL cholesterol, and triglycerides, and also administers a cytomegalovirus human immune globulin IV therapy x 1 hour. Select the correct codes for the physician's work and the laboratory services.

① Z00.00, 99397, 82465, 83718, 84478, 90291, 96374
② Z00.00, 99397, 80061, 90291, 96374
③ Z00.00, 99397, 36415, J0850, 96365
④ Z00.00, 99397, 80061, 90291, 96365

_____ **17.** A patient has a chronic nonpressure ulcer of the right lower leg with fat layer exposed. During an initial operation, the surgeon prepares the site of the ulcer and uses an allograft to permit healing. Thirty days later, the patient is returned to the OR for a free skin flap. What are the correct codes for the second operation?

① L97.512, 15757
② L97.912, 15757 58
③ L97.912, 15757 59
④ L97.512, 15757 76

____ **18.** A surgeon performs a peritoneoscopy to diagnose reported pain in the right lower quadrant of the patient's abdomen. Based on the findings, the surgeon performs a surgical laparoscopic procedure to remove a follicular ovarian cyst. Is the diagnostic procedure included in the surgical procedure in this case?

① Yes
② No

____ **19.** After seeing the patient in the office, the physician admits her for observation. In the hospital, the physician performs a comprehensive history and examination, decision making of high complexity, and decides to schedule the patient for surgery. What procedure code is appropriate?

① 99220
② 99223 57
③ 99291
④ 99220 57

____ **20.** An obstetrician providing routine antepartum, delivery, and postpartum care performs amniocentesis during the first trimester of the patient's pregnancy. Based on CPT, is this service included in the global obstetric package?

① Yes
② No

Appendix A. ICD-10-CM Diagnostic Coding and Reporting Guidelines for Outpatient Services, 2017

These coding guidelines for outpatient diagnoses have been approved for use by hospitals/providers in coding and reporting hospital-based outpatient services and provider-based office visits. . . .

The terms encounter and visit are often used interchangeably in describing outpatient service contacts and, therefore, appear together in these guidelines without distinguishing one from the other.

Though the conventions and general guidelines apply to all settings, coding guidelines for outpatient and provider reporting of diagnoses will vary in a number of instances from those for inpatient diagnoses, recognizing that:

> The Uniform Hospital Discharge Data Set (UHDDS) definition of principal diagnosis applies only to inpatients in acute, short-term, long-term care and psychiatric hospitals.

> Coding guidelines for inconclusive diagnoses (probable, suspected, rule out, etc.) were developed for inpatient reporting and do not apply to outpatients.

A. Selection of first-listed condition

In the outpatient setting, the term first-listed diagnosis is used in lieu of principal diagnosis.

In determining the first-listed diagnosis, the coding conventions of ICD-10-CM, as well as the general and disease-specific guidelines, take precedence over the outpatient guidelines.

Diagnoses often are not established at the time of the initial encounter/visit. It may take two or more visits before the diagnosis is confirmed.

The most critical rule involves beginning the search for the correct code assignment through the Alphabetic Index. Never begin searching initially in the Tabular List as this will lead to coding errors.

1. **Outpatient surgery**

   When a patient presents for outpatient surgery (same day surgery), code the reason for the surgery as the first-listed diagnosis (reason for the encounter), even if the surgery is not performed due to a contraindication.

2. **Observation stay**

   When a patient is admitted for observation for a medical condition, assign a code for the medical condition as the first-listed diagnosis.

   When a patient presents for outpatient surgery and develops complications requiring admission to observation, code the reason for the surgery as the first reported diagnosis (reason for the encounter), followed by codes for the complications as secondary diagnoses.

B. Codes from A00.0 through T88.9, Z00–Z99

The appropriate code(s) from A00.0 through T88.9, Z00–Z99 must be used to identify diagnoses, symptoms, conditions, problems, complaints, or other reason(s) for the encounter/visit.

C. Accurate reporting of ICD-10-CM diagnosis codes

For accurate reporting of ICD-10-CM diagnosis codes, the documentation should describe the patient's condition, using terminology which includes specific diagnoses as well as symptoms, problems, or reasons for the encounter. There are ICD-10-CM codes to describe all of these.

D. Codes that describe symptoms and signs

Codes that describe symptoms and signs, as opposed to diagnoses, are acceptable for reporting purposes when a diagnosis has not been established (confirmed) by the provider. Chapter 18 of ICD-10-CM, Symptoms, Signs, and Abnormal Clinical and Laboratory Findings Not Elsewhere Classified (codes R00–R99) contains many, but not all codes for symptoms.

E. Encounters for circumstances other than a disease or injury

ICD-10-CM provides codes to deal with encounters for circumstances other than a disease or injury. The Factors Influencing Health Status and Contact with Health Services codes (Z00–Z99) are provided to deal with occasions when circumstances other than a disease or injury are recorded as diagnosis or problems.

F. Level of detail in coding

1. **ICD-10-CM codes with 3, 4, 5, 6, or 7 characters**
   ICD-10-CM is composed of codes with 3, 4, 5, 6, or 7 characters. Codes with three characters are included in ICD-10-CM as the heading of a category of codes that may be further subdivided by the use of fourth, fifth, sixth, or seventh characters to provide greater specificity.

2. **Use of full number of characters required for a code**
   A three-character code is to be used only if it is not further subdivided. A code is invalid if it has not been coded to the full number of characters required for that code, including the seventh character extension, if applicable.

G. ICD-10-CM code for the diagnosis, condition, problem, or other reason for encounter/visit

List first the ICD-10-CM code for the diagnosis, condition, problem, or other reason for encounter/visit shown in the medical record to be chiefly responsible for the services provided. List additional codes that describe any coexisting conditions. In some cases the first-listed diagnosis may be a symptom when a diagnosis has not been established (confirmed) by the physician.

H. Uncertain diagnosis

Do not code diagnoses documented as "probable," "suspected," "questionable," "rule out," or "working diagnosis" or other similar terms indicating uncertainty. Rather, code the condition(s) to the highest degree of certainty for that encounter/visit, such as symptoms, signs, abnormal test results, or other reason for the visit.

Please note: This differs from the coding practices used by short-term, acute care, long-term care, and psychiatric hospitals.

I. Chronic diseases

Chronic diseases treated on an ongoing basis may be coded and reported as many times as the patient receives treatment and care for the condition(s).

J. Code all documented conditions that coexist

Code all documented conditions that coexist at the time of the encounter/visit, and require or affect patient care treatment or management. Do not code conditions that were previously treated and no longer exist. However, history codes (categories Z80–Z87) may be used as secondary codes if the historical condition or family history has an impact on current care or influences treatment.

K. Patients receiving diagnostic services only

For patients receiving diagnostic services only during an encounter/visit, sequence first the diagnosis, condition, problem, or other reason for encounter/visit shown in the medical record to be chiefly responsible for the outpatient services provided during the encounter/visit. Codes for other diagnoses (e.g., chronic conditions) may be sequenced as additional diagnoses.

For encounters for routine laboratory/radiology testing in the absence of any signs, symptoms, or associated diagnosis, assign Z01.89, Encounter for other specified special examinations. If routine testing is performed during the same encounter as a test to evaluate a sign, symptom, or diagnosis, it is appropriate to assign both the Z code and the code describing the reason for the non-routine test.

For outpatient encounters for diagnostic tests that have been interpreted by a physician, and the final report is available at the time of coding, code any confirmed or definitive diagnosis(es) documented in the interpretation. Do not code related signs and symptoms as additional diagnoses.

Please note: This differs from the coding practice in the hospital inpatient setting regarding abnormal findings on test results.

L. Patients receiving therapeutic services only

For patients receiving therapeutic services only during an encounter/visit, sequence first the diagnosis, condition, problem, or other reason for encounter/visit shown in the medical record to be chiefly responsible for the outpatient services provided during the encounter/visit. Codes for other diagnoses (e.g., chronic conditions) may be sequenced as additional diagnoses.

The only exception to this rule is that when the primary reason for the admission/encounter is chemotherapy or radiation therapy, the appropriate Z code for the service is listed first, and the diagnosis or problem for which the service is being performed listed second.

M. Patients receiving preoperative evaluations only

For patients receiving preoperative evaluations only, sequence first a code from subcategory Z01.81, Encounter for pre-procedural examinations, to describe the pre-op consultations. Assign a code for the condition to describe the reason for the surgery as an additional diagnosis. Code also any findings related to the pre-op evaluation.

N. Ambulatory surgery

For ambulatory surgery, code the diagnosis for which the surgery was performed. If the postoperative diagnosis is known to be different from the preoperative diagnosis at the time the diagnosis is confirmed, select the postoperative diagnosis for coding, since it is the most definitive.

O. Routine outpatient prenatal visits

See Section I.C.15. Routine outpatient prenatal visits.

P. Encounters for general medical examinations with abnormal findings

The subcategories for encounters for general medical examinations, Z00.0-, provide codes for with and without abnormal findings. Should a general medical examination result in an abnormal finding, the code for general medical examination with abnormal finding should be assigned as the first-listed diagnosis. A secondary code for the abnormal finding should also be coded.

Q. Encounters for routine health screenings

See Section I.C.21. Factors influencing health status and contact with health services, Screening.

Source: Section IV, *ICD-10-CM Official Guidelines for Coding and Reporting*, http://www.cdc.gov/nchs/icd/icd10cm.htm.

Appendix B. CPT Modifiers: Description and Common Use in Main Text Sections

Code	Description	E/M	Anesthesia	Surgery	Radiology	Pathology	Medicine
22	Increased procedural services	Never	Yes	Yes	Yes	Yes	Yes
23	Unusual anesthesia	Never	Yes	—	—	—	Never
24	Unrelated E/M service by the same physician or other qualified health care professional during a postoperative period	Yes	Never	Never	Never	Never	Never
25	Significant, separately identifiable E/M service by the same physician or other qualified health care professional on the same day of the procedure or other service	Yes	Never	Never	Never	Never	Never
26	Professional component	—	—	Yes	Yes	Yes	Yes
32	Mandated services	Yes	Yes	Yes	Yes	Yes	Yes
33	Preventive services	Yes	Never	Yes	Yes	Yes	Never
47	Anesthesia by surgeon	Never	Never	Yes	Never	Never	Never
50	Bilateral procedure	—	—	Yes	—	—	—
51	Multiple procedures	—	Yes	Yes	Yes	Never	Yes
52	Reduced services	Yes	—	Yes	Yes	Yes	Yes
53	Discontinued procedure	Never	Yes	Yes	Yes	Yes	Yes
54	Surgical care only	—	—	Yes	—	—	—
55	Postoperative management only	—	—	Yes	—	—	Yes
56	Preoperative management only	—	—	Yes	—	—	Yes
57	Decision for surgery	Yes	—	—	—	—	Yes
58	Staged or related procedure or service by the same physician or other qualified health care professional during the postoperative period	—	—	Yes	Yes	—	Yes
59	Distinct procedural service	—	Yes	Yes	Yes	Yes	Yes
62	Two surgeons	Never	Never	Yes	Yes	Never	Yes
63	Procedure performed on infants less than 4kg	Never	Yes	Yes	Yes	—	Yes
66	Surgical team	Never	Never	Yes	Yes	Never	—
76	Repeat procedure by same physician or other qualified health care professional	—	—	Yes	Yes	—	Yes
77	Repeat procedure by another physician or other qualified health care professional	—	—	Yes	Yes	—	Yes
78	Unplanned return to the operating/procedure room by the same physician or other qualified health care professional following initial procedure for a related procedure during the postoperative period	—	—	Yes	Yes	—	Yes
79	Unrelated procedure or service by the same physician or other qualified health care professional during the postoperative period	—	—	Yes	Yes	—	Yes
80	Assistant surgeon	Never	—	Yes	Yes	—	—
81	Minimum assistant surgeon	Never	—	Yes	—	—	—

Key: Yes = commonly used   — = not usually used with the codes in that section
                              Never = not used with the codes in that section

(continued)

Code	Description	E/M	Anesthesia	Surgery	Radiology	Pathology	Medicine
82	Assistant surgeon (when qualified resident surgeon not available)	Never	—	Yes	—	—	—
90	Reference (outside) laboratory	—	—	Yes	Yes	Yes	Yes
91	Repeat clinical diagnostic laboratory test	—	—	Yes	Yes	Yes	Yes
92	Alternative laboratory platform testing	—	—	Yes	Yes	Yes	Yes
95	Synchronous telemedicine services rendered via a real-time interactive audio and video telecommunications system	Yes	—	—	—	—	Yes
99	Multiple modifiers	—	—	Yes	Yes	—	Yes

Key: Yes = commonly used   — = not usually used with the codes in that section
                              Never = not used with the codes in that section

NAME _____

CODING QUIZ: ICD-10-CM

1.	①	②	③	④	21.	①	②	③	④
2.	①	②	③	④	22.	①	②	③	④
3.	①	②	③	④	23.	①	②	③	④
4.	①	②	③	④	24.	①	②	③	④
5.	①	②	③	④	25.	①	②	③	④
6.	①	②	③	④	26.	①	②	③	④
7.	①	②	③	④	27.	①	②	③	④
8.	①	②	③	④	28.	①	②	③	④
9.	①	②	③	④	29.	①	②	③	④
10.	①	②	③	④	30.	①	②	③	④
11.	①	②	③	④	31.	①	②	③	④
12.	①	②	③	④	32.	①	②	③	④
13.	①	②	③	④	33.	①	②	③	④
14.	①	②	③	④	34.	①	②	③	④
15.	①	②	③	④	35.	①	②	③	④
16.	①	②	③	④	36.	①	②	③	④
17.	①	②	③	④	37.	①	②	③	④
18.	①	②	③	④	38.	①	②	③	④
19.	①	②	③	④	39.	①	②	③	④
20.	①	②	③	④	40.	①	②	③	④

NAME _____

CODING QUIZ: CPT and HCPCS

1.	①	②	③	④	**21.**	①	②	③	④
2.	①	②	③	④	**22.**	①	②	③	④
3.	①	②	③	④	**23.**	①	②	③	④
4.	①	②	③	④	**24.**	①	②	③	④
5.	①	②	③	④	**25.**	①	②	③	④
6.	①	②	③	④	**26.**	①	②	③	④
7.	①	②	③	④	**27.**	①	②	③	④
8.	①	②	③	④	**28.**	①	②	③	④
9.	①	②	③	④	**29.**	①	②	③	④
10.	①	②	③	④	**30.**	①	②	③	④
11.	①	②	③	④	**31.**	①	②	③	④
12.	①	②	③	④	**32.**	①	②	③	④
13.	①	②	③	④	**33.**	①	②	③	④
14.	①	②	③	④	**34.**	①	②	③	④
15.	①	②	③	④	**35.**	①	②	③	④
16.	①	②	③	④	**36.**	①	②	③	④
17.	①	②	③	④	**37.**	①	②	③	④
18.	①	②	③	④	**38.**	①	②	③	④
19.	①	②	③	④	**39.**	①	②	③	④
20.	①	②	③	④	**40.**	①	②	③	④

NAME _____

CODING QUIZ: ICD-10-CM AUDITING LINKAGE AND COMPLIANCE

1.	①	②	③	④	11.	①	②	③	④
2.	①	②	③	④	12.	①	②	③	④
3.	①	②	③	④	13.	①	②	③	④
4.	①	②	③	④	14.	①	②	③	④
5.	①	②	③	④	15.	①	②	③	④
6.	①	②	③	④	16.	①	②	③	④
7.	①	②	③	④	17.	①	②	③	④
8.	①	②	③	④	18.	①	②	③	④
9.	①	②	③	④	19.	①	②	③	④
10.	①	②	③	④	20.	①	②	③	④

NAME _____

CODING NOTES

NAME _____

CODING NOTES

NAME _____

CODING NOTES

NAME _____

CODING NOTES

NAME _____

CODING NOTES

NAME _____

CODING NOTES